The
Infertility
Answer
Book

BRETTE MCWHORTER SEMBER
Attorney at Law

SPHINX® PUBLISHING
AN IMPRINT OF SOURCEBOOKS, INC.®
NAPERVILLE, ILLINOIS
www.SphinxLegal.com

First Edition: 2005

Published by: Sphinx® Publishing, An Imprint of Sourcebooks, Inc.®

Naperville Office
P.O. Box 4410
Naperville, Illinois 60567-4410
630-961-3900
Fax: 630-961-2168
www.sourcebooks.com
www.SphinxLegal.com

This publication is designed to provide accurate and authoritative information in regard to the subject matter covered. It is sold with the understanding that the publisher is not engaged in rendering legal, accounting, or other professional service. If legal advice or other expert assistance is required, the services of a competent professional person should be sought.

From a Declaration of Principles Jointly Adopted by a Committee of the American Bar Association and a Committee of Publishers and Associations

This product is not a substitute for legal advice.

Disclaimer required by Texas statutes.

Library of Congress Cataloging-in-Publication Data
Sember, Brette McWhorter, 1968-
  The infertility answer book : the complete guide to your family-building choices with fertility and other assisted reproduction technologies / by Brette McWhorter Sember.-- 1st ed.
      p. cm.
  Includes index.
  ISBN-13: 978-1-57248-531-0 (pbk. : alk. paper)
  1. Adoption. 2. Infertility--Treatment. 3. Fertilization in vitro. 4. Human reproductive technology. 5. Pregnancy--Complications. I. Title.

HV875.S39 2005
618.1'78--dc22
                                                    2005021260

Printed and bound in the United States of America.

Dedication

This book is dedicated to my own two beautiful children who came to us after struggles with infertility. They are my joy. My thanks, as always, goes to my husband who supports me in all of my projects and makes me laugh and see the light in the world.

I would also like to thank my own wonderful doctor, Dr. Maria Corigliano, who not only helped us conceive our children, but brought them both into the world with love and skill.

Contents

SECTION I: ASSISTED REPRODUCTION

Understanding Your Condition
What Technology Can Do for You
What Technology Cannot Do for You
Understanding Terminology
Finding Medical Professionals You are Comfortable With
Success Rates
Your Right to ART
Initial Visit
Setting Limits
Privacy
Your Rights as an ART Patient
Weighing Technology vs. Adoption
Weighing the Use of Donors
Ethical Considerations
HIV and Assisted Reproduction
Dealing with Risks
Fertility Specialist Questionnaire

SECTION II: ADOPTION

Affording Adoption
Agency Evaluation Questionnaire
Attorney Evaluation Questionnaire

Home Studies
Consent
No Consent Needed
Notice
Timing of Consent
Consent Procedures
Revocation
Adoption Court Procedures
Postplacement
Birth Certificates
Adoption Financial Credits
Family Leave
Insurance and Planning for the Future

Deciding to Adopt a Stepchild
Qualifications to Adopt
Notice or Consent
Preadoption Procedures
Second-Parent Adoption Process

Public Agencies
Agency Liability
Private Agency Adoption
Interstate Issues
Ethnic Concerns

Introduction

So you want to have a family. There are many ways to create a family. In fact, there are more options available now than ever before. Rapid advancements in reproductive technology have created many possibilities for parents who want to raise a child that is genetically linked to them. These new technologies, such as insemination, surrogacy, embryo adoption, egg donation, and evolving possibilities like cloning or nuclear transfer, allow parents to be connected to a baby from conception. Singles or couples who want to become parents can choose one of the many kinds of adoption—stepparent, domestic agency adoption, international adoption, or independent adoption.

This book is your guide through the many family-building options available. Some people begin building a family with certain ideas about what choices they will consider, while others are unsure of what their options are and how they work. Whether you have a few distinct possibilities you are considering or whether you are still exploring all the options, this book helps you understand how each process or procedure works and explains how to make a child part of your family. This book takes a careful look at the legal procedures and requirements involved in family-building options and helps you understand what steps are necessary to make the child of your heart your legal child.

It is important to note that while this book strives to give you up-to-date legal information, laws are constantly changing. It is essential that you check with an attorney so you can get the most up-to-date information. It is also important to talk with an attorney so you can get personal legal advice based on your individual circumstances.

This book also helps you consider what you are and are not comfortable with and helps you evaluate the options. The book is filled with links to more information available online and an extensive resource list that will help you find books, magazines, organizations, and websites that can offer more information and answer questions.

Section I focuses on assisted reproduction. Chapter 1 helps you understand and evaluate reproductive technology and make informed choices and decisions that are right for you. Chapter 2 addresses the emotional and psychological concerns of ART. The cost of fertility treatments is always a concern. Chapter 3 discusses various options that can help defray these costs. Chapter 4 focuses on single-parent ART considerations. Chapter 5 deals with same-sex couple assisted reproduction. Chapter 6 focuses on insemination, or sperm donation, and some of the issues that surround the use of donor sperm. Chapter 7 looks at egg donation, while Chapter 8 discusses embryo donation (also known as embryo adoption). Chapter 9 talks about the costly and controversial assisted reproductive treatment of surrogacy.

Chapter 10 examines emerging technologies such as cloning. Cryopreservation, or the freezing of eggs, sperm, and embryos, is the focus of Chapter 11. Chapter 12 discusses the issues involved in raising a child who was created using assisted reproductive technologies. Chapter 13 addresses issues about deciding to adopt.

Section II deals with adoption, from the legal process to the many different adoption possibilities. Chapter 14 guides you through the adoption process and explains how adoption works, while Chapter 15 discusses the many options and considerations that are part of the adoption process. The legal procedures and the process you must go through to become an adoptive parent will be covered in Chapter 16. Chapter 17 explains stepparent, or second-parent, adoptions. Chapter 18 examines adoption through a domestic agency, then Chapter 19 deals with international adoption.

Chapter 20 discusses independent (or parent-initiated) adoption when the adoptive parents locate a birth mother without the help of an agency.

Chapter 21 focuses on the ever more commonplace single-parent adoption. Chapter 22 deals with same-sex couple adoption. Chapter 23 discusses how to cope with adoption and handle the bumps along the road, and Chapter 24 is about raising an adoptive child.

The goal of this book is to present you with information so that you can make an educated choice about how you would like to become a parent. Many couples or singles approach family building with the certainty that they want to use assisted reproduction and then later change their minds and consider adoption. The opposite also happens—prospective parents choose adoption, but then change their minds and use assisted reproduction. This book will guide you through all the choices and help you no matter what path you decide to pursue, now or in the future.

Building a family is one of the most important decisions you will make in your life. This book will help you as you consider and select the avenue that will work best for you.

Choosing Assisted Reproduction or Adoption

You have picked up this book because you are considering advanced fertility procedures or adoption to help you build your family, or you at least want some information about those choices. Choosing to seek help or get information about the options available to help you build or create a family is a big step. It can be frightening to face the wide choices in front of you and difficult to understand what your rights are and how to navigate through the processes.

Some couples instantly know which they are interested in pursuing—advanced fertility treatments or adoption. Other couples reach this crossroads and simply do not know how to proceed. Spend some time reading about the options available to you and familiarize yourself with the legal procedures. If you want information on medical procedures, how they work, and how they affect you, check the appendices for books and websites that can educate you about this.

It can be difficult to compare adoption with fertility treatments because they are completely different approaches to family-building and also because there are so many types of fertility treatments and adoption options. Use these basic questions to help you get a feeling for which path feels more comfortable for you.

- How important is it that you or your spouse be biologically related to your child?
- Would you be comfortable raising a child from another country or one who looks physically very different than you do?
- How important is it that your child live with you beginning in the newborn period?
- How willing are you to undergo medical procedures and tests in the hopes of building a family?
- How much money do you have available to spend on family-building? (See the chart on the following page to understand costs.)

Approximate Costs of
Advanced Fertility Treatments vs. Adoption:

Fertility Treatments:

Donor Insemination: $500 per cycle
Egg Donation: $7500 per cycle
Embryo Donation: $3000 per cycle
Surrogacy: $25,000 to $50,000

Adoption Procedures:

Foster Care Adoption: $2500
Domestic Agency Adoption: $4000 to $30,000
International Adoption: $10,000 to $40,000
Domestic Parent-Facilitated or Independent Adoptions: $8000 to $30,000

Advanced Assisted Reproduction

Pros:

- You can create a child who is related to you or your partner or spouse.
- One of you may be able to carry the pregnancy and give birth to the baby.
- No one will know you have had assistance in conceiving, unless you choose surrogacy.
- You may be able to conceive quickly and with minimum intervention, giving you a child very soon.
- The birth parents will not have any ongoing role in your child's life and will remain anonymous (unless you choose embryo adoption, see Chapter 8).
- There are no court procedures to go through (unless you use surrogacy).

Cons:

- Drug therapies and medical procedures can be uncomfortable and time consuming.
- You must rely on a physician and possibly donors to help you become pregnant or a parent.
- You pay whether you conceive or not (unless you take advantage of packages with guarantees).
- You may need to use someone else's genetic material to create a child and you may not have a lot of control over who the donor is.
- If you do a lot of cycles or have to try many different procedures, fertility costs can be greater than adoption costs.

Adoption

Pros:

- Depending on the type of adoption you choose, you can be almost certain that a child will be placed with you.
- The costs for an adoption are more fixed than they are for fertility procedures where you have additional costs every time you do another cycle or try a new procedure.
- You may be able to see or meet your child before you make the final decision to adopt him or her.
- You do not have to go through the agonizing waiting process each month of finding out if you're pregnant.
- You know that you've done something wonderful for a child that needs a home.

Cons:

- It will be obvious to others that you have adopted.
- It is very unlikely that you will be able to adopt a newborn.
- If you adopt internationally you may have very little information about your child's family history and medical background.
- The birth parents may want to meet you and have ongoing contact with your child.
- You must pass a home study in order to be allowed to adopt and you must go through a court process to legally adopt your child.
- It is more expensive to pay for an adoption than it is to pay for one or two less invasive fertility procedures.

Section I
Assisted Reproduction

Chapter 1

Understanding & Evaluating Reproductive Technologies

Reproductive technology has reached a point where there are many options available to help you become parents. These options have given couples a lot of freedom, opened the doors to wonderful new possibilities, and created many families. When you are considering using reproductive technologies to help you become a family, there are a lot of points to weigh and a lot of information to gather.

Understanding Your Condition

If you are considering assisted reproduction, it is important that you come into the process with a good understanding of why natural conception is not working for you and what conditions or problems have brought you here. Understand what your doctor thinks is realistic for you and your partner and what the odds are for you with the different types of treatment. Many times, doctors cannot give you a complete answer as to why you cannot conceive without assistance, but it is important to arm yourself with whatever knowledge is available.

In general, it is best to try the least-invasive procedures first, if they provide real hope for you. This book talks mainly about fertility treatments that involve input from other people, but many couples are able to conceive using their own genetic material. There are many good treatments that are noninvasive, including drug therapies. Be sure to explore all of the options available to you and understand what could or could not work not before progressing to more invasive and complicated treatments.

What Technology Can Do for You

Technology can help you or your partner become pregnant; provide you with genetic material to create a baby if your body cannot do so itself; or, allow you to work with another woman to gestate your pregnancy. These options can seem staggering. Most people begin at the bottom of the totem pole with the least expensive and invasive options and work their way up to more expensive and complicated procedures.

What Technology Cannot Do for You

While technology can offer you new ways to become parents, it cannot change the basic facts of your circumstance. It cannot help you cope with the emotional effects of being unable to conceive on your own. Technology cannot erase basic biological facts. Technology can provide you with a baby, but it cannot always provide you with a baby that is genetically linked to both you and your partner. This can be a big stumbling block for many couples.

For many couples, it is possible to have a child that is a biological child of one of the parents, while using donor material for the other. This raises the issue of whether you and your partner are comfortable with all this implies—having a child who will resemble one of you but not the other; having a child who has an unknown or unidentified parent; and, the inevitable emotional fallout as you process these facts and live with them in the years to come.

Understanding Terminology

The assisted reproductive field is filled with acronyms for different types of procedures. Following are some definitions of these terms that will be used throughout the book.

ART—assisted reproductive treatment. This is the medical assistance you receive as you try to conceive.

GIFT—gamete intrafallopian transfer. Eggs (either belonging to the intended mother or obtained through donations) are retrieved from the ovaries and placed in the fallopian tubes with sperm. Conception occurs in a natural location, but allows physicians to carefully choose the genetic material available.

ICSI—intracytoplasmic sperm injection. A single sperm is injected into an egg and the egg is then implanted into the intended mother.

IVF—in vitro fertilization. Eggs are fertilized with sperm outside of the mother and embryos are implanted into her uterus.

IUI—intrauterine insemination. Ovulation is induced in the woman and sperm is then inserted into the uterus.

ZIFT—zygote intrafallopian transfer. Eggs are retrieved from the mother or donor and inseminated. The zygote or young embryo is then implanted into the fallopian tube.

Other terms you may come across include the following:
- *gamete.* This refers to sperm or eggs—the building blocks of a baby.
- *induced cycle.* Ovulation that is induced by medication.
- *natural cycle.* Ovulation that occurs without medication or medical intervention.
- *oocytes.* An egg before maturation.

Finding Medical Professionals You are Comfortable With

As you begin your journey into the world of assisted reproduction, the most important thing you can do is select doctors and clinics that you are comfortable with. The process you are entering is very stressful and emotional. If you are working with providers who are not sensitive to your needs or who you just feel uncomfortable with, the entire process will be more difficult for you.

The first place to start is with your OB/GYN. Get a referral to a fertility

From the Expert

For more information about options and available treatments, see:

www.fertility neighborhood.com/ content/treatment_options/ default.aspx

and

www.babycenter.com/ refcap/preconception/ fertilityproblems/4093.html

specialist. If you are not happy with that referral, ask for another. If there is a medical school in your area, call them and ask if the school is involved in a clinic in your area. Talk to other couples you know who have used assisted reproduction about what doctors and facilities they have used.

Before visiting a specialist or clinic, call and ask if the providers are board certified or board eligible in gynecology and obstetrics as well as in *reproductive endocrinology*. Fertility specialists should be certified in both of these areas. If the clinic has an IVF lab, ask if it is accredited by the College of American Pathologists (whether or not you plan on using IVF). All labs of any kind must be accredited under the federal *Clinical Laboratory Improvement Amendment* (CLIA). Ask if the physicians are members of the American Society of Reproductive Medicine. Most reputable clinics also have the following specialists on staff:

- reproductive immunologists;
- embryologists;
- reproductive urologists;
- andrologists; and,
- genetic counselors.

When meeting with a medical provider, there will be much information you need to gather from him or her. Use the checklist on page 15 to help the process move smoothly.

Success Rates

When you interview clinics, it is important to ask about *success rates*. This will let you know how successful the clinic is at producing pregnancies. The most important success rates are the number of take-home babies per year and the number of live babies born per cycle. (The number of pregnancies can be a deceiving statistic because many may fail early in the pregnancy.)

Keep in mind that some clinics may not have high success rates because they focus on difficult-to-treat problems or because they use last ditch methods that may be a couple's only hope. Make sure you understand why a clinic's numbers are what they are.

Your Right to ART

Fertility clinics cannot turn you away because of a disability or discriminate against you because of your race or ethnic background. At the time this book was written, a case was being heard in Colorado about a blind woman who was required to show a clinic that she was able to care for a child before they would continue her IVF treatments. The court will consider whether the *Americans with Disabilities Act* prohibits this kind of discrimination. Clinics that receive federal funds may also violate the *Rehabilitation Act* if they treat those with disabilities differently than other patients.

> **From the Expert**
> You can check a clinic's success rates online at:
> **www.cdc.gov/needphp/ drh/arts/index.htm**

Initial Visit

When you visit a fertility specialist, it is important to bring medical records, test results, and reports with you. Both partners (if you are part of a couple) should be at the first visit so that both can meet the doctors and ask questions. Ask yourselves if you feel comfortable with the people you meet there and with the general atmosphere. You also need to be frank with yourselves about what you can afford. Try to get clear answers about success rates. Evaluate what you are told with a critical eye.

When you first meet with a fertility specialist, it is a good idea to have something to write on and to bring a list of questions with you. You can use the list at the end of this chapter. You are entitled to ask the staff anything you want. There are no restrictions on the types of questions you can ask. It is important to not only get hard information about the clinic, their success rates, the doctor's qualifications, and the treatments available, but also to get an impression as to whether this is someone you are comfortable working with and relying upon.

You can expect to complete a family medical history and your personal medical histories (with an emphasis on your reproductive health), and perhaps undergo an exam and tests at your first visit.

Setting Limits

Most couples enter the world of assisted reproduction slowly—first with fertility drugs and then gradually moving on to other procedures. When you first begin to work with medical assistance to get pregnant or have a child, it is important to have a frank discussion with your partner about what types of medical assistance you are comfortable with. This is not a topic that normally comes up in most marriages, but once you begin to work with fertility specialists, a whole world of possibilities opens before you. You may not know how your spouse feels about sperm donors, egg donors, and surrogates.

Realize that what you think you know about your feelings and preferences now may change. If you move through different procedures with no success, you may feel that that the desire to have a child is more urgent than any objections you might have had earlier to certain types of fertility assistance.

Privacy

You and your partner will also have to make some choices about who you will tell about your ART procedures and what information you are willing to share with family, friends, and so on. You are not obligated to tell anyone, but most couples find they need the support that friends and family can provide.

Because ART procedures are medical procedures, they are protected by the *Health Insurance Portability and Accountability Act* (HIPAA). Your doctor or insurance company cannot give out any medical information (verbally or in writing) about you without your consent. Information can be shared without your consent to coordinate treatment between doctors (such as if you are working with an a reproductive endocrinologist and a reproductive surgeon) or to obtain payment from insurance. Your information cannot be given to your employer or used in a marketing or advertising campaign without your consent. In order for information to be released to your insurance company, you need to sign a onetime waiver stating that you want your health insurance company to be billed and that you agree to have information released to them.

If you want your spouse or partner to be able to have access to your records (or even to be able to call in with a question on your behalf), tell the office staff you would like to give written permission for this. Although the law says that a family member involved in your care can have access to your records, doctors are very careful about this. If you have an unmarried partner, it is essential that you give permission for him or her to access your records.

HIPAA also gives you the right to see your own medical records, obtain a copy of them, and get a report about when and with whom your health information was shared. You have the right to require doctors, clinics, and hospitals that treat you to make corrections to your records or to at least note that you disagree with information included in your record.

> **From the Expert**
>
> If you believe that your medical privacy rights have been violated, contact the Department of Health and Human Services at 866-627-7748 or:
>
> **www.hhs.gov/ocr/hipaa**

Your Rights as an ART Patient

This may be the first time in your life you have had to seek serious medical intervention. It is important to know what your rights are.

Who is the Patient

Most people enter ART with a partner or spouse. When you approach the treatment with a partner, it feels to you as if both of you are the patient, since you are trying to create a child together. While your doctors may talk to you both together and treat you the same way, only the person who is receiving medical treatment from the provider is the patient. Because of privacy laws, if a woman is the one receiving treatment and her husband calls the clinic to get a test result or ask a question, the clinic is not supposed to release the information to him.

The way around this is to sign a release form that will be kept in your file. This will authorize the clinic to speak to both of you about any treatment, test results, or procedures at any time. Your clinic will have a form they will want you to complete, but they may not offer it automatically — you will probably have to ask for it. Giving your partner access to your treatment will help make this a joint venture and will also allow you the convenience of not having to make every phone call yourself.

Informed Consent

When you receive medical treatment, you must provide informed consent. This means that you must agree to the treatment after all the risks and benefits have been explained to you. Fortunately, in ART, your care providers will probably spend a lot of time talking with you about treatments, risks, and possible outcomes. If at any point you feel you do not have enough information to make a decision or if you feel confused about something, speak up and ask for more information. Always be sure to ask about risks and possible outcomes for you as well as for your child.

It is also important that you take the time to educate yourself about your condition and treatments. Spend some time doing Internet searches and reading articles so that when you see your provider, you are armed with some knowledge and are better able to ask questions. (See the resources provided in the Appendices for further information.)

Second Opinions

You always have the right to a second opinion, and most insurance companies will pay for one. A second opinion is a good idea when you have been given bad news or when an invasive treatment is recommended. Do not ask your current doctor for a recommendation about who to see — he or she is likely to send you to someone with a similar viewpoint. Instead, contact your insurance company and ask for names of other specialists or contact the national organization for the type of specialist you are seeing.

Refusing Treatment

You have the absolute right to refuse medical treatment and can walk out of any doctor's office, clinic, or hospital at any time. Refusing treatment is sometimes referred to as leaving *against medical advice* (AMA). You can change your mind about treatment, decide you want a second opinion, or feel that you need more time to think about something.

The one caveat that is involved with ART is that women are at the mercy of their cycles, so if you are scheduled for an IVF treatment but need time to think about it, you may miss your window of opportunity for that month. Additionally, if you have medical insurance that is paying for your care, and you refuse a recommended treatment, the insurance company may not pay for any complications or problems that result from your refusal of treatment.

Experimental Treatments

Because the ART field is constantly evolving, there may be new treatments available to you that have not been fully tested, proven, or reviewed. If you are considering an experimental treatment, find out what other options you have and compare them and their success rates with the experimental treatment. Some couples go to experimental treatments when everything else has failed, while others are anxious to try new things that may have better or faster results than more traditional treatments.

Educate yourself about the treatment—its costs, its risks, and its benefits. Ask a lot of questions and get information about what kind of testing it has undergone and what bad results have occurred. Find out how experienced the practitioner is with the treatment. Get information about costs up front. Your insurance company is unlikely to pay for experimental treatments, but it cannot hurt to ask. Some experimental treatments are funded by universities or other groups that reduce or remove any cost to you.

Weighing Technology vs. Adoption

There comes a point, once you have not been successful with fertility drug treatment, that you must choose a path. You must decide whether you want to pursue becoming a family through adoption or becoming a family through assisted reproduction. It is important to understand that no decision you make at this crossroad has to be the final word. It is possible to pursue both options at the same time and then, if one works, give up on the other. It is also possible to begin down one path only to change your minds and pursue the other choice. In other words, you are not making a final, irrevocable decision no matter what you start to do.

Some couples simply know which path they will pursue. Others need to think about the possible outcomes, financial costs, and emotional costs of both choices. There is no right or wrong answer.

Weighing the Use of Donors

When you enter into ART, you probably do so planning to use your own genetic material to conceive a child. But some couples are unable to do so and must use donor material. Choosing to use donor material involves an acceptance of what you are giving up. You are giving up your dream of having a child that is genetically related to you and your partner.

Many couples are able to have a child that is genetically related to one of them, but not the other. In this instance, you and you partner must be able to live with this knowledge. Some couples experience real problems over this. Seeing your wife carry a child that another man's sperm helped to create or carrying a baby that was created with another woman's egg can be a difficult burden. Some people feel jealous of the parent who will be genetically related, resentful that they are unable to genetically participate, or worried that somehow the child will not be as much theirs.

It is very important to consult with a counselor when making these decisions. Conceiving via ART can be a long and arduous journey. You could be carrying this pain for a long time. It is important to resolve these feelings, because if you do successfully conceive, you want to be able to parent with a loving and open heart.

Ethical Considerations

Depending on which ART you use, you may be faced with decisions that are ethical as well as practical. These can include what you will do with extra eggs that have been harvested or frozen embryos that you have not used. Once you have reached the decision that you will not be using this material, you are faced with a choice of what should happen with it. These decisions are highly personal, but boil down to three options — donate the genetic material to another couple or person who can use it; donate it to research; or, have it destroyed. Each option involves personal, religious, moral, and emotional issues. There are no laws governing what should happen to this material, but there can be disputes between couples about how to dispose of this material.

To get details on your state insurance laws, check with your state insurance department.

HIV and Assisted Reproduction

It used to be thought that a person with HIV should not use ART because of the risks involved to the other partner. It was feared that if the person providing the sperm is HIV positive, there would be a potential danger of contracting the virus to the woman carrying the pregnancy. New techniques that allow *sperm washing* have substantially reduced these risks. The key in any ART procedure involving HIV is complete disclosure. For example, if you are using a surrogate and the partner providing the sperm is HIV positive, it is important that the surrogate know this and be fully informed of any risks involved.

Dealing with Risks

Because you are considering cutting edge medical technology, it is important that you come to a clear understanding of the risks posed to you and your partner, as well as to your possible children. Medical risks should be discussed thoroughly and completely with your medical care providers. Do not allow your providers to assume you understand risks. Ask to have them spelled out. There are risks of infection and other problems from surgical procedures, as well as risks posed by fertility drugs used to stimulate ovulation, by pregnancy itself, and by other procedures you may encounter.

In addition to medical risks, you also face legal risks. When you are dealing with your own genetic material, the legal implications are not as great. However, when you begin to consider and use procedures that involve donated eggs, sperm, or zygotes (embryos), the legal risks become much larger.

It is imperative that you work closely with a reproductive rights attorney who has experience reviewing and drafting contracts for donations and surrogacy. Do not assume you can do this on your own. This book is designed to point out the important issues, considerations, and questions that should come up, but is not designed to allow you to do it yourself. Because you are dealing with your legal rights as a parent, you want an expert on your side.

NOTE: *To find a reproductive law attorney, contact your local or state bar association for a referral.*

Fertility Specialist Questionnaire

Name of Specialist_____

Date of Interview_____

Questions:

❑ Where did you go to medical school and complete your residency?

_____

❑ How many years have you been a fertility specialist?_____

_____

❑ How many reproductive endocrinologists are on staff?_____

_____

❑ Will we work with you or several doctors?_____

_____

❑ Is there someone on call after hours?_____

_____

❑ Are you affiliated with a hospital?_____

_____

❑ What insurance plans do you accept?_____

_____

❑ Are payment plans an option?_____

_____

❑ How much will the proposed treatment cost?_____

_____

❑ What does that include?_____

_____

❑ What is your practice's number of take-home babies (babies that are born and go home with their intended parents)?_____

_____

❑ What treatments and services do you offer?_____

_____

❑ Can you provide referrals should we require other treatments?

_____

continued

❏ What support services do you offer?_____

❏ What is your rate of live babies per cycle?_____

❏ Is your lab accredited by the American College of Pathologists or the Joint Commission on Accreditation of Health Care Organizations?_____

❏ Do you report results to the Centers for Disease Control (CDC)?_____

❏ How long will it take to diagnose our problem?_____

❏ What tests and procedures do you use to perform the diagnosis?_____

❏ If necessary, can you help us access a donor egg, sperm, or embryos?

❏ How will we communicate with you through the process?_____

Chapter 2

Coping with ART

The decision to use assisted reproduction can be a difficult one for many people. Some people come to ART after months or years of trying to conceive on their own. Some people learn very quickly that they need assistance conceiving. No matter how long you've been dealing with fertility issues, it is still a complicated and emotional decision to choose to use assisted reproduction. You have to admit, at least to yourselves, that you need help and intervention to accomplish your dream of having a child. It can be truly devastating to come to terms with the fact that you probably aren't going to be able to conceive a child on your own without some kind of medical intervention.

Taking the very private decision to have a baby and seeing it become clinical, medical, and financial can be very painful. Because this is such a difficult decision, it is important to understand how to cope and live with your ART procedures.

Deal with Emotions
The ART process is very emotional and that is often amplified if you're taking hormones that make you even more emotional. You've got to have a plan for dealing with your ups and downs. Be prepared to face depression and euphoria, often in the same week. Some couples find that it is helpful to talk with a therapist to help them deal with the emotions they face. Some clinics have nurses on staff who are trained to help patients deal with the emotional issues. Others have psychologists or psychiatrists

on staff who can help you. Some clinics even have special relaxation and de-stressing programs at the clinic to help patients learn to manage the overwhelming feelings the process often creates.

In addition to your spouse and medical support staff, you might find you want to reach out to other couples who are going through similar feelings and problems. Find a support group and just go and listen for a while and see if you want to participate.

Talk with your spouse about how much you want to reveal to other people about what you're going through. Some people share all the details with family and friends. Others are more private. It is interesting that when a couple is trying to adopt that other people find it to be fascinating and wonderful, but when a couple is trying to use ART to conceive a baby it somehow is shameful and not something that should be shared.

> **From the Expert**
>
> Contact *RESOLVE,* The National Infertility Association, at 888-623-0744 for information about local support groups and online groups or visit the website at:
>
> **www.resolve.org**

Making Time for ART

ART requires a time commitment from you. You must take drugs, have regular appointments, and make room in your life for the emotions that the drugs and procedures bring with them. It is not a small commitment. As you begin the ART journey, the commitment may be small, but the farther you go, the bigger the commitment becomes. It can be difficult to juggle a job with this focus.

If you're worried about how all of your medical tests, appointments, procedures, and meetings are going to impact your job and if you don't have a lot of sick time available to use for this, you have the option of taking time off under the federal *Family and Medical Leave Act* (FMLA). The law allows you to take time off, unpaid, for your own medical needs, or to care for a family member. You are entitled to up to twelve weeks total per year and you can arrange this time any way you need to. You might decide to take off three months while you're doing IVF, or you might want to take off one week a month, or you could decide you want to cut your hours in half while you're dealing with ART.

You are eligible for leave under the FMLA if you work for a public agency (federal, state, or local) or for a private employer with fifty or more employees and have been employed there at least twelve months and worked at least 1250 hours in the last twelve months. When possible, you must provide your employer with thirty days notice, but if you suddenly find you just can't cope with going into work and it's all too much for you, your employer can accommodate you.

Under the FMLA, your employer must keep your health benefits in place (but you may have to pay premiums while you are out) and must restore you to original job or to an equivalent job with equivalent pay when you return. Your employer cannot penalize you for taking the leave or allow it to affect any of your benefits. If you return to work and your employer has taken away some of your job responsibilities or cut your hours, this would be a violation.

If you and your spouse work for the same employer, you are entitled to a total of twelve weeks unpaid FMLA leave divided between both of you in a twelve-month period to care for your child. So for example, you could take ten weeks and your spouse could take two weeks. Your leaves can be taken simultaneously. Spouses who work for different employers are entitled to each take the full FMLA twelve weeks. If you experience any problems with your FMLA request, contact the Department of Labor at **www.dol.gov**.

Some states have family leave laws as well, so check with your human resource department to find out if you are entitled to state family leave time as well.

Keeping Your Relationship Stable

The ups and downs of ART can make even the happiest people cranky, hysterical, and self-absorbed. It's important to remember that even though you may both be experiencing things differently physically speaking, you are emotionally in this process together. Rely on each other and support each other as you go through the difficult and amazing days ahead. Making a baby together is a wonderful, amazing process, but it can be easy to lose sight of that when you're juggling drugs, appointments, and weighing heavy decisions such as donors.

Make time for each other and for your life as a couple. Find a way to do fun things that help you block out all the ART stuff you're dealing with. Try to make time for spontaneous affection, even though you have a clinical schedule to follow.

Live Your Life

Although you may find a lot of your time and thoughts are taken up with medical concerns, it is important that you keep it from becoming all-consuming. Spend time with friends, make time for things you enjoy, and continue to find pleasure in your life. It's difficult to make long range plans at this point in your life since every cycle you're hoping that you'll have life-changing news, but at some point you have to realize you can't just put your entire life on hold and have to move forward with your career, your social life, and your interests. You can always make room in your life for a baby, but it is almost impossible to fill a big gaping hole when you plan around a baby that hasn't materialized yet.

ART requires a time commitment from you. You must take drugs, have regular appointments, and make room in your life for the emotions that the drugs and procedures bring with them. It is not a small commitment. As you begin the ART journey, the commitment may be small, but the farther you go, the bigger the commitment becomes. It can be difficult to juggle a job with this focus.

Chapter 3

Affording Fertility Treatments

The decision about whether to use fertility treatments and how far you're willing to go is deeply linked to cost for many couples. It can be easy to get in too deep and spend more than you affordably can on fertility treatments. No one plans to go broke using assisted reproduction, but it happens in a gradual way. You pay for the drugs and tests and those don't get you results. So you escalate to insemination and then decide to try one in vitro cycle, then another, and another. If that gets you nowhere, you may move on to donors and then to a surrogate. It's a slippery (and expensive) slope once you start down it.

Insurance

Your first step to managing the financial aspect of your treatments is to explore what your insurance will cover and what it will not. In most states, insurance companies are not required to provide coverage for infertility procedures. However, coverage is normally provided for diagnosis and treatment if there is an underlying medical cause for the infertility, such as endometriosis.

To determine if you have coverage for infertility treatment, ask your employer for a copy of your health insurance policy contract. If your contract does not specifically exclude infertility treatment, then it is covered. If it mentions infertility treatments, read it carefully to see what, if anything, it does cover. It might, for example, cover diagnosis of infertility problems, but not actual treatment.

You also need to check your prescription drug coverage and find out which fertility drugs are covered and which are not. If your policy appears to provide coverage, but payment is denied for a treatment you or your spouse undergo, you can appeal the decision. Check your contract for details on how this is done. Denials are usually made because infertility is not an illness, the treatment was not medically necessary, or the procedure or treatment is experimental. None of these are valid reasons for denial of coverage. A letter from your doctor is a helpful piece of evidence to use in an appeal.

Additionally, you may be able to prove that the denial of coverage violates the *Americans With Disabilities Act* (ADA). A 1998 Supreme Court case, *Kraul v. Iowa Methodist Medical Center*, held that infertility meets the requirements of the ADA. You need to speak to your attorney to discuss this option.

Be sure to check your coverage for a lifetime maximum for fertility treatments. Some policies put a cap on how much they will pay in total for one patient over a lifetime.

Insurance Coverage

The following states are currently the only ones that mandate insurance coverage for infertility.

Arkansas. HMOs exempt from this law. Coverage for IVF with a two-year history of infertility or medical conditions causing it. Coverage is provided only if a patient's eggs are being fertilized by her husband's sperm. There is a lifetime cap on these benefits.

California. Coverage if infertility of one year or infertility creating medical conditions exist. GIFT is covered, but in vitro is not mandated for coverage. Coverage is required to be available (meaning there is an extra cost), but is not required to always be included in policies.

Connecticut. Coverage must be available, but does not have to be included in policies unless chosen. Includes diagnosis, treatment, and in vitro. Available for women who have been infertile for one year.

Hawaii. Provides a one-time-only in vitro benefit if there is a five-year infertility history and the patient's eggs are fertilized with her spouse's sperm.

Illinois. Diagnosis and treatment provided after one year of infertility. A wide varieties of treatment is covered including IVF, GIFT, and ZIFT.

Maryland. Coverage required for IVF, but HMOs are exempt. The patient's eggs must be fertilized with the spouse's sperm.

Massachusetts. Diagnosis and treatment covered for women who have been unable to get pregnant in a one-year period. Includes insemination, IVF, GIFT, ZIFT, and other treatments. Coverage for surrogacy and cryopreservation is optional.

Montana. HMOs required to provide coverage for infertility, but the law is vague as to what this entails.

New York. Covers diagnosis and treatment of infertility, but does not cover IVF.

Ohio. HMOs required to provide coverage for infertility. There is a $2000 cap if the infertility does not have a stated medical cause.

Rhode Island. Provides coverage for diagnosis and treatment of infertility.

Texas. Provides coverage for diagnosis and treatment including IVF. The patient's eggs must be fertilized by the spouse's sperm.

If you are married, be sure to check both your policy and your spouse's policy, since once of you might have more extensive coverage. If this is the case, the spouse with the extensive policy would add the other spouse onto the policy and go to a family policy instead of an individual one.

From the Expert

Read a listing of major companies that offer infertility coverage online at:

**www.inciid.org/
printpage.php?cat=
insurance101&id=16**

A list of current state insurance coverage and exclusions is available at:

**www.fertilityjourney.com/
financialAspects/
insurancelaws/index.asp**

This might cost more in employee contributions, but if the coverage is better, this investment will pay off. Remember that once your child is born you will need a family policy anyhow, so you're simply taking that step a little sooner than you would have had to anyhow. (To get details on your state insurance laws, check with your state insurance department.)

Thinking About Costs

Because fertility treatments can be so costly and because many people do not have insurance coverage for it, it is important to give some serious thought to your financial situation and how you are going to approach treatments. Fertility treatments are an investment. They are an investment that does not pay you back in dollars, but pays you back in happiness if you are successful. However, they are a high-risk investment because 50–60% of couples who use infertility treatments are successful, which means 40–50% are unsuccessful. It is essential that you talk with your doctors about your chances, your situation, and the specific procedures you are contemplating. It is also important to talk with your doctors about your age and whether spending a few months or a few years saving money before beginning treatment is an option for you. Some couples are able to take a year and squirrel away everything they can in order to afford the procedures they need, while others know the clock is ticking, or simply feel that they are emotionally unable to put off their dream.

Getting a Handle on Costs

To be able to make a decision about what exactly you can afford and how many cycles you can pay for, you have to get a grip on exact costs. While this book offers estimated costs for different advanced procedures, you need to talk with your doctors to find out what the costs will be in your case. Ask about costs for:

- the procedure itself;
- lab work before and after the procedure;
- prescriptions before and after the procedure;
- ultrasounds and other tests before and after the procedure;
- fees for specific physicians that are not included in the procedure costs; and,
- anesthesia.

Guarantees

Some clinics offer special programs that include guarantees. For example, one such program guarantees that you will get pregnant in three IVF cycles if you are of a certain age and meet certain conditions. If you do the treatment and don't get pregnant, you get a refund for all of your costs for the failed procedures. These types of guarantees can sound good, but it's important to shop around and compare costs. If you do get pregnant, these programs might have a higher cost per cycle than other programs because in effect the people who get pregnant are carrying the financial burden for the people who are unsuccessful. On the other hand, if you do three cycles and get no results, this could work out to be a very good deal for you.

Medical Spending Accounts

There are two types of medical spending accounts that can be used to pay for fertility expenses.

Health Savings Account (HSA)

These are special medical savings account that can be created by anyone who has a health insurance plan with a minimum family deductible of

$2000 or minimum individual deductible of $1000. You can contribute up to $2600 for individuals or $5150 for families per year into the account. The money is placed in the account tax-free and must be used to pay medical expenses. Money you do not use each year remains in the account and can be used in later years. Withdrawals not used for health care costs are taxed and subject to a 10% penalty. The key to using an HSA is good record keeping. Whenever you pay for a medical expense, you must keep the receipt so that you have proof the funds were used for medical expenses. Talk with your financial advisor for more information on setting up one of these accounts.

Flexible Spending Account (FSA)

A flexible spending account is set up by your employer. You contribute pretax funds to the account and then are reimbursed from the account for health care expenses (including any health insurance premiums you pay as well as health care expenses that are not covered by your insurance plan and over the counter mediations) that you have during the year. Because you do not pay tax on the reimbursement funds, the money is tax-free. Depending on your income, you may be able to contribute between $2000 and $5000 a year to the account. If you do not use the money in the account in the calendar year, you forfeit the balance.

> ### From the Expert
> Use the online FSA calculator to find out if one makes sense for you:
> **www.principal.com/ grouplh/selffunded/ fsacalculator.htm**
>
> Get details about what expenses an FSA can be used for at:
> **www.irs.gov/ publications/p502/ index.html**

Financing Fertility

If you don't have enough savings to cover the costs of your infertility treatments right now, you don't have to give up. Many fertility clinics offer payment plans and financing options. Payment plans allow you to space out your payments over a period of time instead of paying cash up front. Financing plans are usually through a third party financing company that the clinic has established a relationship with. These financing plans usually offer interest rates slightly lower than you could obtain on your own and may be an affordable option for some couples. Repayment terms range from a year to sixty months. When evaluating a financing plan make sure there are no balloon payments (large payments required at certain points in the lifetime of the loan), the interest rate is competitive with other unsecured loans, that you understand exactly what the payments will be, you know whether you can increase the amount of your loan to cover future treatments if the treatment you have planned does not work, and if you can repay the loan before the scheduled end of the repayment plan. If you have a financial advisor, you should consult with him or her to discuss whether some of the other options in this chapter would work better in your situation.

If these options don't work for you, there are other paths you can take, but it is important that you seriously think through the implications. Some people consider the following:

- borrowing money from family or friends;
- refinancing their home;
- taking out home equity loans;
- selling their home;
- changing jobs to a job with better ART coverage;
- considering a part-time job that offers insurance;
- joining a fertility drug study;
- donate eggs in exchange for treatment;
- taking loans against retirement plans; and,
- taking loans against life insurance.

These are desperate measures that some people feel are justified. It is important that you consider your financial future though. If you sell your home and your treatments are successful, how will you buy another one? If you take a loan against a retirement plan, how will you repay it and manage the expense of raising a child if your treatments are successful?

And what if your treatments are unsuccessful and you want to be able to afford adoption or live a comfortable child-free life? These are important considerations that must be thought through.

If you are a state or government employee, you can access your Deferred Compensation Plan. You may be able to withdraw funds from the account to pay for treatments, although it is sometimes questionable whether fertility treatments meet the test required (it must be "an unforeseeable emergency").

Taxes

You may be entitled to deduct some of your fertility treatment costs on your income tax return as medical expenses. You can deduct medical expenses that are over 7.5% of your adjustable gross income. Talk with your tax preparer to find out if you can deduct your expenses. If you think you may be able to deduct these expenses, start a file now and keep all of your receipts from doctor visits, lab work, prescriptions, and tests. You can also keep a mileage log and deduct mileage to and from medical appointments as well as trips to the drugstore.

Chapter 4

Fertility for Singles

It is no longer uncommon for a single person to want to conceive a child. While some people may not be comfortable with your choice, it is a choice that is available to you, and is one more and more singles are finding to be the right one for them.

Finding Medical Providers

Your primary concern must be to find a doctor or clinic that is welcoming to singles. Most fertility specialists are used to dealing with couples, but more and more have now had the opportunity to work with an unmarried person. Be upfront about your marital status and the fact that is just you who will be the baby's parent. You may want to call ahead and ask if the clinic welcomes singles, which can help you avoid an uncomfortable situation.

Some doctors and clinics will be more welcoming than others. Sperm banks, for example, are quite accustomed to single women using their services while it is more unusual for a single man to use a surrogate or for a single woman to use an egg donor. The bottom line though is that you have the right to create a child in any way that works for you.

Discrimination

Discrimination against singles by doctors and clinics is much less common than it was in the past. It is also often veiled. A physician might tell you that in his or her opinion, you have little chance of conceiving and that the clinic will not take your case, when you haven't been given any solid reasons why you can't conceive. Unfortunately, there is no antidiscrimination law that covers this, so if you believe you've been treated unfairly, your best course of action is to first find a new doctor and secondly to report the incident to your state medical board ethics committee.

Considerations

When planning to become a single parent, it is important to consider all of your options and all of the ramifications of your choices. Many, many children are raised by single parents and without question, single parents can definitely raise happy and healthy children. When deciding to become a single parent, it is important to have a good support system in place. You need friends and family you can rely upon for emotional and practical help. It is a good idea to take a close look at your financial situation and your plan for the future. Raising a child is an expensive proposition and some single parents find that it is difficult to continue to work full-time or afford day care costs. It most definitely can be done though, so it is a good idea to create a financial plan for your new family.

As a single parent, you may also wish to consider purchasing life and disability insurance. Disability insurance will provide protection for your family should you become unable to work and support your family. Life insurance provides a measure of security for your family should you die unexpectedly. It is also a good idea to have a will drawn up and name a guardian who will care for your child in the event that something should happen to you.

Single parents must be prepared to deal with ignorance and insensitivity as they raise their children alone. "Where's his father?" and "What do you mean she only has one parent?" are examples of the types of questions you may encounter. It's also important to give some thought to how you will tell your child about his or her origins and other parent.

Chapter 5

Gay and Lesbian Assisted Reproduction

It is common for gay couples to become families using assisted reproduction. Today more physicians and clinics are welcoming to gay and lesbian couples than ever before. It is probably more commonplace for lesbian couples to seek assistance (normally through a sperm bank) than it is for gay male couples to seek egg donors or surrogates, so you can expect the path to be easier for lesbians than for gay male couples.

Finding Doctors and Clinics

There is no protection from discrimination for gays and lesbians seeking assisted reproduction. Conversely, there is no law that prevents gay couples from using ART and there are many clinics and doctors that have no problem working with gay couples. Seek out a gay-friendly clinic. Call ahead and ask if gay couples are welcome. If you know other gay or lesbian couples who used ART, find out where they went or what health care providers they used.

From the Expert

For information on arranging for a private donor, see *Gay Family Options* at:
www.gayfamilyoptions.com

or *Rainbow Flag Health Services* at:
 www.gayspermbank.com

For more resources, visit *Prospective Queer Parents* at:
 www.queerparents.org

Legal Parents

In states where gay marriages or unions are recognized (such as Massachusetts, Vermont, and Connecticut) as well as states like California where domestic partners are given many rights, a child that is born to one partner during the marriage, union, or domestic partnership is legally the child of the other partner. This means that you do not need to do a second-parent adoption procedure in these states (although it may still be a good idea because if you move to another state that does not recognize and uphold your state's laws, you will want to be sure that legal parentage cannot be questioned).

> **From the Expert**
>
> For information about finding gay-friendly clinics, see **www.lesbianhealthinfo.org/ask-the-dr/answer.htm**

> **From the Expert**
>
> For information about a gay-friendly sperm bank, see **www.gayspermbank.com**

If you do not live in a gay marriage state or if you want to be sure to cover all of your options, the partner who does not carry the child (or does the initial adoption if you conceive via a surrogate) will need to do a second-parent adoption procedure (see Chapter 17).

Discrimination

In California, a lesbian sued her fertility clinic when they refused to treat her because of her sexual orientation. The California appeals court ruled that this was unlawful discrimination under California state law and that physicians cannot deny patients treatment because of their sexual orientation. California and fourteen other states (including Vermont, New Hampshire, Massachusetts, New Jersey, Connecticut, District of Columbia, Hawaii, Illinois, Maine, Maryland, Minnesota, New Mexico, Rhode Island, and Wisconsin) have civil rights laws that ban discrimination against gays in public accommodations, including health care services. If you live in one of these states and are discriminated against, report it to your state attorney general's office.

Gay couples may come up against discrimination not only from clinics, but from insurance companies. Some insurance companies define infertility as the inability to get pregnant after six months of traditional intercourse,

> **From the Expert**
>
> For information about gay surrogacy options, see **www.growinggenerations.com**

thus defining gays and lesbians as people who do not qualify for coverage for infertility treatment. At this point there is no recourse for this kind of discrimination, other than individual lawsuits against insurance companies, which have yet to be successful.

Chapter 6

Insemination

Insemination is a procedure in which sperm is inserted into a woman's body to attempt conception. There are a variety of ways insemination can occur. The simplest way is to use the male partner's sperm and insert it through the vagina. The insemination process is used so that the sperm can be sorted and the most viable sperm can be used.

When using sperm that comes from the male partner, the legal issues and problems are minimal. The couple is receiving medical assistance with their own genetic material. This chapter focuses on the issues surrounding the use of *donor sperm*, which is sperm that does not belong to the partners of a potential single mother.

Laws

There are no laws prohibiting the use of insemination by married or unmarried couples or by singles, so anyone is free to pursue this option. Before choosing donor insemination, it is important that a couple knows the cause of their infertility and their chances of pregnancy without donor insemination.

When a woman who is married gives birth, the child is legally her husband's. So if a married couple uses a sperm donor, the husband is the legal father and no steps are necessary to ensure this. Some states require the husband to consent in writing to the insemination.

The areas that do not require the husband's consent include:
- Arizona
- Delaware
- District of Columbia
- Georgia
- Hawaii
- Indiana
- Iowa
- Kentucky
- Louisiana
- Maine
- Maryland
- Massachusetts
- Michigan
- Mississippi
- Nebraska
- New Hampshire
- North Dakota
- Pennsylvania
- Rhode Island
- South Carolina
- South Dakota
- Tennessee
- Utah
- Vermont
- West Virginia

In the following states, laws remove any rights of donors:
- Alabama
- California
- Colorado
- Connecticut
- Idaho
- Illinois

- Kansas
- Minnesota
- Missouri
- Montana
- Nevada
- New Hampshire
- New Jersey
- New Mexico
- North Dakota
- Ohio
- Oregon
- Texas
- Virginia
- Washington
- Wisconsin
- Wyoming

Types of Sperm Donors

There are two types of sperm donors—known and unknown.

Known Donors

A *known donor* is often a friend or family member of the couple or potential single mother. Using a known donor has advantages and disadvantages. The main advantage is you know exactly where the sperm came from, what the person's traits are, what his personality is like, and details about his medical history. You also have the ability to have ongoing contact with him after the pregnancy so that the child can someday meet and possibly have a relationship with him. Another advantage of postpregnancy contact is that you will have access to any medical information that comes to light after the insemination—for example, if the donor is diagnosed with diabetes or heart disease.

The disadvantages of a known donor are the emotional complications that can ensue. If the donor is a family member or close friend, the parents could come to resent his presence in the child's life or the donor could come to feel resentful about his small role in the child's life. Knowing the donor and having contact with him could cause confusion for the child (although in most cases this is not a huge issue—nontraditional family ties are not so unusual these days).

If you use a known donor, you should still enlist the assistance of fertility specialists and clinics who can make sure the procedure is done appropriately and can put some safeguards in place. Even though you know the donor, you will want to be sure his sperm is tested for disease. Certain testing can take several weeks.

Some women or couples choose to do home inseminations. While the cost can be greatly reduced, the effectiveness may be decreased. If you do choose to do your own, make sure you use an insemination agreement. (See Appendix B for a sample agreement.)

> ### From the Expert
> For information on home insemination, visit:
> **http://homeinseminations. homestead.com/index.html**
> or
> **www.fertilityplus.org/faq/ homeinsem.html**

It is important for legal reasons as well as medical reasons to have the insemination performed by a physician. In some states, the rule about the married woman's husband being the legal father of a child produced through insemination only applies if the insemination was performed by a licensed physician.

Additionally, it is important that all the parties involved in the insemination procedure—the woman, the donor, and the woman's partner if one exists—obtain counseling. This will not only help the parties work through any problems they have with the procedure, but also will help ensure that problems will not appear in the future. Counseling ensures that everyone involved is certain about the decision and is emotionally able to handle its repercussions.

Agreements with Known Donors

Even though you have some kind of relationship with the donor, it is essential that you sign a legally binding insemination agreement. (See Appendix B for a sample Insemination Agreement.) It is important that you use a reproductive law attorney to draft an agreement that will meet the requirements of your state.

The agreement will have the donor give up all rights to custody or visitation with the child. This is essential so that he does not later change his mind and decide to seek custody. The woman receiving the sperm gives up all rights to seek anything from the donor, including child support.

If the woman receiving the donation has a partner, it is important that the partner sign the agreement and indicate his or her consent to the procedure as well. If the partner is her husband, this will further ensure that the child will be legally his. Information about nonmarried partners is provided later in this chapter.

Unknown Donors

Unknown donors are generally located through a *sperm bank*. Sperm banks pay donors for their sperm and carefully screen donors and their sperm for medical conditions and disease.

Certain states specifically require HIV screening of donor sperm. These states include:

- Arizona
- California
- Connecticut
- Delaware
- Florida
- Idaho
- Illinois
- Indiana
- Iowa
- Kentucky
- Louisiana

- Maryland
- Michigan
- Montana
- North Carolina
- North Dakota
- Ohio
- Oklahoma
- Rhode Island
- Virginia
- West Virginia
- Wisconsin

NOTE: *If your state does not specifically require HIV screening, you will want to be sure your clinic does it anyway.*

The sperm is frozen and preserved until testing is complete. The sperm bank makes sure that donors and the women who receive the donations receive counseling to help them cope with the decision. The woman using the sperm is charged a small fee—often between $200 and $400 for the sperm, not including the cost of the insemination procedure.

Sperm banks offer profiles of donors that include medical history, ethnic background, physical attributes, mental abilities, personality traits, and photos. Clients of the sperm bank can choose a donor that is physically similar to them in some way or who meets other criteria they have.

There is no government regulation of sperm banks in the US, although four states do license sperm banks: California, Maryland, Massachusetts, and New York. Some sperm banks are accredited by the *American Association of Tissue Banks* (AATB) but most are not. Additionally, the *American Society of Reproductive Medicine* (ASRM) has guidelines that the banks should follow. Some banks may say they meet or exceed the AATB guidelines, but this does not mean they are actually accredited by AATB, so be sure to pin this down. State health departments also offer certification of sperm banks, but you should be most concerned with AATB certification.

In 2005, the FDA created new rules that prohibit gay men from anonymously donating sperm if they have had male partners within the last five years. The new law also requires sperm banks to test donors and donated sperm for HIV, hepatitis B, hepatitis C, syphilis, and other diseases, as well as sexually transmitted infections like chlamydia and gonorrhea. Sperm banks are required to ask donors about their risk factors for such diseases. This rule doesn't apply when the sperm is being transplanted into the donor's partner or for people who are repeat anonymous sperm donors.

The facility should have guidelines that provide for:

> **From the Expert**
>
> Contact the *American Association of Tissue Banks* at:
>
> **www.aatb.org**
>
> and the *American Society of Reproductive Medicine* at:
>
> **www.asrm.org**

- obtaining a complete medical history from the donor;
- personal interviews with all donors;
- freezing sperm for six months to allow for complete testing of the donor and to do freeze tests on the sperm;
- careful record keeping;
- tracking of the number of pregnancies per donor;
- limiting of the number of pregnancies per donor;
- physical exams and blood tests for all donors for many diseases including HIV, Tay Sachs, Sickle Cell, etc.;
- medical history going back four generations whenever possible;
- genetic and chromosomal analysis;
- ruling out mental health issues;
- shipping of sperm using nitrogen;
- the use of cryoprotectants that do not use chicken egg extract (due to possible allergies); and,
- set minimum number of sperm per sample.

The sperm bank will provide the donor agreement and will ensure that both you and the donor are protected from future problems with custody and support. However, it is a good idea to have your own attorney read any agreement you are asked to sign.

Donors are not notified when their sperm is used, so they are very distant from the insemination process. Donors are paid a small amount for each donation they provide.

If you are ordering sperm from a sperm bank for home insemination, the sperm bank requires a physician's authorization to release it because donor sperm is considered a medical substance. Thus, it is necessary to see a doctor and have him or her agree to or approve your plans for home insemination through a sperm bank.

Legal Parents

As previously mentioned, when a married woman receives donor sperm and the procedure is performed by a physician, her husband is the legal parent of the child. If a donor agreement is used, the sperm donor has no rights to the child and cannot be held liable for support.

If an unmarried heterosexual couple uses insemination, the male partner will need to legally adopt the child after the birth using a second-parent adoption process. (See Chapter 17 for more information.) The mother will be the only legal parent of the child until this point. The donor's right will be terminated by the donor agreement.

If a single woman uses insemination, she is the sole parent of the child. The donor's rights are terminated by the agreement.

If a gay female couple uses insemination, the woman who gives birth is the sole legal parent of the child. The partner can adopt the child using a second-parent adoption procedure if it is permitted in their state. A gay male couple might use insemination coupled with egg donation and a surrogate. (See Chapter 8 for more information on egg donation; Chapter 9 for information on surrogacy.)

> ### From the Expert
> The *American Society of Reproductive Medicine* has a free booklet on insemination available online at:
> **www.asrm.org/Literature/patient.html**

Future Considerations

If you use donor insemination—whether it is from a known or unknown donor—it is important that you gather as much medical information about the donor and his family as you can find. This information will be important for your child.

Many sperm banks make it a condition of donation that the donor's identity can be revealed to children created from his sperm once they become adults. This can be an important policy that will make locating the biological parent easier for your child.

Talking about donor insemination with you child can be challenging, since it is complicated to discuss both in its physical sense as well as in an emotional sense. Be prepared for a lot of questions. Be honest with your child to the point he or she is able to understand. (See Appendix A for resources regarding books for children about insemination.)

Choosing a Sperm Bank
Questionnaire

Name of Agency_____

Name of Contact Person_____

Date of Interview_____

Questions:

❏ How long have you been doing this?_____
_____

❏ Are you licensed or accredited by any state or organization?_____
_____

❏ Do you follow ASRM guidelines?_____
_____

❏ What procedures are used to test the health of the donors and the sperm?_____
_____

❏ What other screening do you do with donors?_____
_____

❏ How long do you keep records?_____
_____

❏ Do you follow ASRM record-keeping guidelines?_____
_____

❏ Can clients select the donor themselves?_____
_____

❏ What donor information is available?_____
_____

❏ Are current and baby pictures available from each donor?_____
_____

❏ Are personal statements available from donors?_____
_____

❏ Is the health of the donors monitored on an ongoing basis after donations are made?_____
_____

❏ Do you track the number of pregnancies per donor? *(This is important so that there are not too many children from any one donor. Large numbers of offspring from any one donor would increase the risk that these children might someday meet and reproduce without realizing they are siblings.)*_____

_____

❏ Is donor sperm available for a second child?_____

_____

❏ Do you act as a middleman should the child, once he or she is grown, wish to contact the donor?_____

_____

❏ Is stem cell storage available from the umbilical cord?_____

_____

❏ Do you store cells from the donor that can later be tested if necessary?

_____

❏ Do you provide contact information so that children can contact their biological fathers?_____

_____

Chapter 7

Egg Donation

Egg donation is an option that allows a woman to carry a pregnancy, even if she does not produce eggs or produce eggs that result in pregnancy. A donor provides the eggs. The eggs are then inseminated by the woman's partner, or by a donor, and implanted in the intended mother. Some women prefer this option over adoption because not only does it allow them to have a child that is genetically related to their partner, but also because they are able to experience the pregnancy and control the environment in which the child is gestated.

Some women feel uncomfortable with the process, as if it somehow highlights their biological imperfections. Others feel uncomfortable at the notion of their partner's sperm mixing with eggs from another woman. Ultimately, using a donor is a personal choice that must be carefully considered.

Finding a Donor

Some women who need an egg donor are able to ask a family member or friend for the donation. Relatives, such as a sister or cousin, are sometimes preferred so that the child will carry similar genes as the mother.

Other women prefer to use donors who have no connection to them. These donors may be known or unknown. Some clinics have egg donor programs, where women donate eggs for compensation. Other clinics encourage women who are undergoing ART to donate extra eggs they create during the process for use by another infertile woman (often offering the donor some kind of reduced fee arrangement for her own

> **From the Expert**
>
> Search for egg donation agencies by state online at:
>
> **www.everythingsurrogacy. com/cgi-bin/main.cgi? eggagency**

treatment). It is also possible to locate a donor on your own, by placing ads in newspapers (particularly college newspapers) and reaching an agreement on your own with a donor.

There are a limited number of egg donors available (since the process is so arduous), and not a wide selection of donors to choose from if you are choosing a donor from those available in a clinic. If you are locating your own donor, your selection may be even smaller since few women are willing to go through the process. When you do locate an egg donor, make sure you that you obtain a complete medical history from your donor since this will be important for your child's medical care.

Donation Process

Egg donation is more complicated than sperm donation. Eggs cannot be frozen effectively yet (or, at least, it is not yet considered to be completely reliable by most specialists in this area, although technology is rapidly advancing), so the donor and the woman receiving the donation must have their cycles adjusted so that the egg can be removed from the donor and implanted into the intended mother. Both must take medication to adjust their cycles. The donor must undergo a minor surgical procedure to extract the egg, causing the risk of complications such as infection or possible damage to her ovaries.

Before the procedure, the donor is tested for various diseases. However, because the egg donation must occur immediately, eggs, unlike sperm, cannot be tested extensively.

It is highly recommended that both the donor and recipient, as well as their partners, undergo counseling to help them deal with the hormonal fluctuations of the process, as well as the emotional consequences.

Once the eggs are harvested, they are fertilized using an IVF technique or a GIFT or ZIFT technique. Fertilized eggs are implanted in the intended mother and she carries the pregnancy.

Another type of egg donation may soon be available. While it has only been successful in animals to date, it may soon be possible to transplant *ovarian tissue* (parts of the ovary) from one woman to another. This would allow an infertile recipient to create eggs using donor material. The eggs would have genetic material from the donor only, but would be grown and fertilized inside the recipient's body. Should this procedure become more common, recipients should be certain they have an agreement with the donor that any children resulting from the donation will be the intended mother's.

The FDA created new regulations in 2005 that requires tissue banks to test donors and donated eggs for HIV, hepatitis B, hepatitis C, syphilis, and other diseases, as well as sexually transmitted infections like chlamydia and gonorrhea. Tissue banks are required to ask donors about their risk factors for such diseases. This rule doesn't apply when the egg is being transplanted back into the donor (such as when you use IVF, or if you are using a surrogate who is using her own eggs for the procedure).

> **From the Expert**
>
> For more information on the donation process, see: **www.infertilitydocs.com/ infertility/egg_donation.html**

Cost

The cost for one egg donation cycle is approximately $15,000 and includes the costs for both the donor's and recipient's care and clinic costs. If you are paying your donor additional compensation for her time or discomfort, your costs will be higher. Some donors are paid up to $7500 per cycle. Unlike in adoption or other types of donation, the donor is actually paid for her donation because it is such an arduous procedure and one that carries risks of impacting her future fertility.

Ask the clinic for a breakdown of costs for the following items:
- application and consultation;
- donor screening;
- screening for you and your partner;

- donor reimbursement;
- drugs for donor and yourself;
- ultrasounds and blood tests;
- oocyte retrieval;
- lab procedures;
- implantation of oocytes; and,
- freezing, storage, and thawing of oocytes.

Agreement

It is essential to use a legally binding agreement with an egg donor. It is always best to have a reproductive law attorney draw up the agreement or have your attorney check the agreement provided by the clinic. The agreement is very similar to the one used for insemination donors. Agreements state that the donor gives up all rights to the eggs and any children conceived from them. Donors have no right to custody or visitation and cannot be sued for child support. The agreement will specify that the intended parents will be financially responsible for the entire donation process, including counseling, medical costs, and prescription costs. If the donor is to be paid, the specific amount should be specified.

The donor should be required to provide a complete family medical history. Some agreements may require the donor to provide ongoing health history if conditions develop.

The egg donor, the recipient, and their partners (if any) should sign the agreement. The agreement should also specify that the donor (and her partner if she has one) will take any steps necessary to ensure that the child is legally that of the intended parents. Consent should also be obtained for some of the eggs to be fertilized and then frozen for future use. It important that the donor is fully informed about what is involved in the procedure and all risks that are associated with it.

> ### From the Expert
> View a sample egg donation agreement online from the *American Surrogacy Center* at:
> **www.surrogacy.com/legals/ eggdonationconsent.html**

State Laws

Florida, North Dakota, Oklahoma, Texas, Virginia, and Washington have laws about egg donation that state that the donor gives up her rights to the egg under a valid donation agreement, and therefore, cannot be held responsible for child support and has no right to custody or visitation with any resulting children. Florida specifically allows reasonable financial compensation to the donor. Other states have no laws about egg donation.

There have been cases in both New York and Ohio about ownership of embryos (that have been cryopreserved). In both cases, the intended parent couples divorced and disputed ownership of the resulting embryos or custody of children born from the embryos after the divorce. In both cases, the intended mother (the divorcing wife) prevailed over the man. (See Chapter 11 for more information about cryopreservation and disposition of eggs or embryos after divorce.)

Legal Rights

Once a donor signs a valid donor agreement, she and her spouse (if any) agree to give up all rights to any eggs donated and any children that may result from the donation. The woman who receives the donation will carry the pregnancy. The child she gives birth to is legally hers, and if she is married, her husband is the legal father.

If a single woman receives an egg donation and uses a sperm donation to fertilize the egg, she is the sole legal parent of the child.

If an unmarried couple uses egg donation and the male partner's sperm, the child is legally a child of the mother at birth. The man is not a legal father until a legally binding *paternity acknowledgment* is made (this can often be done by filing paperwork with the state putative father registry) or until a court issues a judgment of paternity. In some states (such as California) paternity can be established prior to birth if there has been adequate prebirth testing that establishes the genetic link.

It is rare for a female homosexual couple to use egg donation, since between the two women there is likely to be one partner who can ovulate without assistance. However, it is an option that is available. The partner who gives birth to the child is the legal parent and the other partner would need to use stepparent adoption to become a legal parent.

Male homosexual couples are more likely to use a surrogate who can provide the egg herself, thus making egg donation an unnecessary step.

Future Contact with the Donor

Most couples who use an unknown donor have no ongoing contact with her. More and more families that use egg donation are open about it with their children. Your donor agreement may specify that the donor is to remain anonymous or it may leave the door open for future contact. Some parents want their children to be able to locate the donor once they are adults.

Donors are usually not told if their donations result in pregnancy, so they do not have the same reactions birth mothers do in adoption situations. Most egg donors are interested in the financial incentives the program offers and are happy to know they are also able to help infertile couples. Donors are not told who gets their eggs, so they remain removed from the process.

Ovarian Tissue Donation

Recently, some ovarian tissue donations have been successful and have resulted in births. If you are considering an ovarian tissue donation, follow the guidelines in the chapter, just as you would for an egg donation.

Choosing a Clinic
Questionnaire

Name of Clinic_____

Name of Contact Person_____

Date of Interview_____

Questions:

❑ Does the clinic have an existing pool of donors?_____

_____

❑ How does the clinic get donors?_____

_____

❑ How are donors compensated?_____

_____

❑ Does the clinic work with recruiters to locate donors?_____

_____

❑ What is the age range of donors?_____

_____

❑ Do donors remain anonymous?_____

_____

❑ Will you work with a donor we bring into the program?_____

_____

❑ How are donors screened?_____

_____

❑ How long is the wait to get a donor?_____

_____

❑ What amount of control do we have over the donor chosen for us?___

_____

❑ Are donors covered by their own or the clinic's health insurance?____

_____

❑ What are your statistics and success rates?_____

_____

❑ Do you meet ASRM guidelines?_____

_____

continued

❏ Is psychological testing done?_____
_____

❏ Will you work with our insurance company?_____
_____

❏ What payments are due at what time and what kind of refund is available if we change our minds?_____
_____

Chapter 8

Embryo Donation

Embryo donation occurs when an egg that has been fertilized and has begun to develop into a baby (sometimes also called a *zygote*—but technically an embryo is a few days older than a zygote) is donated to a mother or couple that did not provide genetic material for the child.

These embryos or zygotes are usually extras that have resulted when other couples have undergone ART procedures. Because these procedures usually produce more zygotes than are safe to implant at once, couples undergoing these procedures often freeze the extras. The original intent may be to save them for later ART cycles if the current one is unsuccessful. The couple may also intend to save them in order to have siblings later.

Although there are many ART couples producing many extra zygotes, few actually donate them to other couples. Once they have gone through the very long and difficult process of ART, these frozen embryos seem very valuable to them and it is difficult to give them away after they worked so hard to create them. Additionally, some couples may feel uncomfortable about donating them and having another couple raise their biological child. Instead, these couples often find themselves more comfortable with a zygote donated to science for research purposes only.

There have been at least fifty-three children born using embryo donation according to a recent survey by the *Embryo Donation Task Force*, and there are over 188,000 frozen embryos in America. Compared to the number of children adopted each year or conceived using other ART, this is very small. However, it is an option to consider and one that may best fit the needs of some couples.

Embryo donation is also sometimes called *embryo adoption*. The terminology used is important because it has implications for the pro-life and pro-choice movements. If it is known as embryo adoption it gives more weight to the argument that embryos are humans. Embryo donation is the term used more often since it is a more neutral term.

When you accept an embryo donation, it is like accepting a child without seeing him or her. You have no idea what you will get—and you also do not know if the embryo will actually implant. It is likely that your child will have siblings in the world that you will never know about, since most embryo donations come from other couples undergoing ART with the purpose of having a child.

Embryo donation has been in the news recently. The federal government invested $1 million in a public awareness campaign to improve awareness about it as an option, while at the same time opposing the use of embryos for research. While this is a political power play, it has helped to bring the issue of embryo donation to the forefront.

Embryo donation has benefits and detriments. The following list looks at its pros and cons.

Embryo Donation

Pros:

- It is much faster than adoption.
- The intended parents completely control the pregnancy.
- The intended mother gives birth to the baby and can nurse.
- Genetic siblings are possible if there are enough embryos from the donor couple.
- The process offers greater privacy than adoption.
- Complete genetic screening is done on the embryos.
- Complete medical information about biological parents is provided.
- You do not have to pay an egg donor or pay for the expenses of a birth mother.
- The legal risk is low since the donor couple never knows about the pregnancy and cannot attempt to get custody of the child or otherwise interfere.

Cons:

- Donors tend to be people who have fertility problems themselves, so the embryos may have some problems.
- There is very little selection or choice since there are few embryos available.
- You cannot meet the biological parents and may not even see a photo of them.
- Donors tend to be older.
- Your child may have full genetic siblings in the world without your knowledge.

From the Expert

You can access a list of clinics that handle embryo donation at:

**www.resolve.org/main/
national/embdon/Resource
Directory.pdf**

From the Expert

Snowflakes is one of the only agencies that handles embryo adoptions in a process similar to traditional adoptions. They can be contacted at:

Snowflakes
*Nightlight Christian
Adoptions*
801 East Chapman
Suite 106
Fullerton, CA 92831
714-278-1020
www.snowflakes.org

For embryo donation information, you can contact *Reprotech* at:
www.reprot.com

National Embryo Donation Center at:
www.embryodonation.org

Finding a Donor

Some clinics arrange embryo donation and match donors and recipients themselves — with attention paid to ethnicity and physical characteristics. Recipients usually do not have the ability to select their donors as they do with other types of donation. The clinic restricts donors to those that are young enough and have no medical conditions or histories that would be of concern. Counseling is recommended for both couples in an embryo donation to make sure that everyone involved understands the process and can handle it emotionally.

The FDA regulations requiring testing of sperm and egg donations for HIV and other diseases also applies to embryo donors, who must undergo these tests before donating embryos for use by other couples.

Embryo Adoption

Another option is an embryo adoption, which is a modified form of embryo donation and is not to be confused with the term of the same name sometimes used for embryo donation. (see p.55.) An outside agency that is not associated with the clinic handles the matching process. Recipients are provided with more information about the donors and counseling and home studies are performed in much the same way they would be in a traditional adoption. Donors have some say in choosing the recipient and also have the option of staying in touch with them and possibly knowing their genetic children at some point down the line.

State Laws

California, Florida, Louisiana, North Dakota, Oklahoma, and Texas have laws permitting embryo donation that make the recipient or recipient couple the legal parent or parents. Florida permits reasonable compensation to the donors. Other states do not have laws about embryo adoption or donation. The process is handled by the contract created by the parties.

The recipient mother or couple is/are the legal parent(s) of a child born through embryo donation or adoption. As soon as the embryo is implanted in the mother, she is its legal parent because under state laws, the woman who gives birth to the baby is its legal mother. Her husband is the legal father, since under state law the husband of a woman who has a baby is its legal father. If she has an unmarried partner he can adopt the child via second-parent adoption. This same procedure applies to gay female couples.

Some couples that accept donations are not comfortable with the lack of law in this area and thus seek to protect themselves by going through an adoption procedure after the child is born, since if DNA tests were ever done, it would prove the child to be the product of the biological donors. It is important to talk to your reproductive rights attorney about how you can best protect your family and follow your state's laws.

Costs

Costs for embryo donation are similar to those for IVF, but there may be additional costs for the donation of the embryo. Costs average $3000 per transfer. If your embryo is being shipped to you, you will have additional shipping

From the Expert

Information about embryo adoption is available through *RESOLVE* (the National Infertility Association) at:
www.resolve.org/main/nati onal/embdon/index.jsp

costs, which run in the hundreds since the embryo must be carefully preserved during the shipping process. The donor couple is not paid for the donation.

Agreement

Generally, there are two separate agreements involved in embryo donation. The donors sign an agreement giving up all rights to the frozen embryos. This could occur years before a recipient is found. Often, this is part of the original contract that the couple signs when they begin ART at the clinic. Most agreements specify what will happen to unused or extra embryos. The recipients sign a separate agreement with the clinic agreeing to accept the embryo and dealing with the medical risk factors involved. Recipients must receive full disclosure of all risks. Donors and recipients usually have no direct contact and are not aware of each other's identity. Be sure to have your reproductive law attorney read any contract from a clinic before you sign it.

> ### From the Expert
> A sample agreement for embryo donation can be read at:
> **www.dreamababy.com/ download_files/Embryo%20 Donation%20Stipulation%20 Agreement.pdf**

The agreement should contain the following:
- a complete release of all rights by the donors;
- a clear explanation of costs;
- a description of what happens if an embryo does not thaw and cannot be implanted;
- an indication that you have received full disclosure and understand the risks involved;
- an agreement as to whether or not you will receive additional donations should they be needed; and,
- a treatment program you will be receiving.

If you are interested in an embryo donation in which the donors are involved in the selection process, you will find that there are no laws governing this process. Agencies that take this approach treat the process as a traditional adoption and have the donor and recipient sign consent forms as they would in a regular adoption.

Issues

There are a lot of issues involved with this type of donation. First is the consideration that if you are trying to conceive, you may not get the best possible results by using an embryo created by another couple that was having trouble conceiving themselves.

Because a number of embryos usually must be implanted in order to achieve one viable pregnancy, couples are faced with the problem of trying to find a donor that can provide more than one embryo or opt to use embryos from several donors simultaneously. Should twins result, they could have completely different genetic parents. Also, the parents would never know which donor couple created the child and could spend an inordinate amount of time looking for characteristics or hints from the children themselves.

Privacy

Another issue involved with embryo donation is privacy. It is possible to keep the fact of the donation to yourselves and not share the information with family and friends. Some people choose not to share this information because they believe their child would be treated differently or that their family and friends would have a negative reaction to the donation. Some family members are unable to let the information go and spend years wondering aloud about the donors and their characteristics. It is, however, important to share the donation with your obstetrician and pediatrician in case there is ever a health issue that could be impacted by the donation fact.

Some parents decide to share information about the donation with their child, while others prefer not to reveal this information. As with adoption, it is a matter of personal preference how much you want to share with your child and what you feel comfortable revealing.

Clinic Evaluation
Questionnaire

Name of Clinic_____

Name of Contact Person_____

Date of Interview_____

Questions:

❑ What kind of release have the donors signed?_____
_____

❑ Do they relinquish all rights to the embryos?_____
_____

❑ How many embryos are available from this couple?_____
_____

❑ Do you ever recommend using a mixture of embryos from different couples?_____
_____

❑ Will I learn the names of the donors?_____
_____

❑ Will the donors learn our names?_____
_____

❑ What information can I learn about the donors?_____
_____

❑ What medical and family history is available?_____
_____

❑ Are photographs of the donor couple available? (*Some recipients like to have photos to show their children or to get a sense of what their baby might look like.*)_____
_____

❑ How do you match donors and recipients?_____
_____

❑ Do we have any say in how the clinic matches donors and recipients?
_____

❏ Does the donor couple have a say in how the clinic matches donors and recipients?_____

❏ What is your success rate with embryo donation?_____

❏ How many embryo donation transfers have you performed?_____

❏ How long have you been performing this procedure?_____

❏ Have any children resulted from embryos from this couple? (*You will want to know if your child has any living siblings.*)_____

❏ Have embryos from this couple been donated to anyone else and will they be in the future? (*You want to be sure that no one else is receiving donations to limit the number of siblings out there in the world for your child.*)_____

❏ What was the age of the donors at the time of donation? (*Younger is better.*)

❏ How long has the embryo been frozen? (*An older embryo may not be as effective as a newer one.*)_____

❏ What kind of treatment did the donating couple undergo?_____

❏ Why did they donate the embryos?_____

❏ Are the eggs and sperm used to create the embryo the donor couple's own or were they donations?_____

❏ If the eggs and sperm used to create the embryo were donations, what information is available about these donors?_____

(continued)

❑ What screening and testing has been done of the donor couple and the donated embryos?_____
_____

❑ If the embryos do not survive thawing, what financial adjustments or refunds are made? (*You want some kind of adjustment.*)_____
_____

❑ What are the total fees for this process?_____
_____

❑ What support services are available?_____
_____

Chapter 9

Surrogacy

Surrogacy is perhaps the most controversial of all ARTs currently available. A surrogate is a woman who agrees to carry a pregnancy for another person or couple. There are two types of surrogacy—one where the surrogate is biologically related to the child and the other where she has no biological connection. In *traditional surrogacy*, the surrogate's own eggs are used and are inseminated with the intended father's sperm. *Gestational surrogacy* occurs when the surrogate is implanted with an embryo created with the intended parents' genetic material or with donor eggs or sperm.

Surrogacy can cost from $25,000 to over $50,000, depending on the difficulty involved with conception, the medical issues present in the pregnancy, and what expenses and costs the intended parents are responsible for under the contract.

Laws Concerning Surrogacy

There is no general legal trend about surrogacy in the United States yet, and states tend to be all over the board. As such, five general categories of how states address surrogacy have developed.

States where it is a crime to pay for surrogacy:
- Michigan
- New Mexico
- New York
- Utah
- Washington

Areas where surrogacy contracts are **unenforceable:** (This means you cannot ask a court to enforce it, however you are free to enter into one, knowing you will not be able to obtain assistance from the court)
- District of Columbia
- Indiana
- Louisiana
- Nebraska
- New York (you are free to enter into an unpaid agreement, but it is a crime to pay for surrogacy)
- North Dakota
- Virginia

States that **recognize** *surrogacy agreements through laws:*
- Arkansas
- Florida (reasonable compensation is permitted)
- New Hampshire
- Nevada
- Tennessee
- Texas
- Washington (you cannot pay for surrogacy, but you can agree to unpaid surrogacy)
- West Virginia

States that have caselaw *about surrogacy:*
- California (permits surrogacy)
- Kentucky (prohibits surrogacy programs and payments, but this is largely unenforced)
- Massachusetts (a recent case encouraged the legislature to enact laws permitting surrogacy)
- Ohio (surrogate who is biologically related must relinquish rights in order for intended mother to become legal parent and the state will not enforce surrogacy contracts)
- Oklahoma (permits surrogacy, but requires the surrogate's husband (if any) to refuse to consent to what is technically considered to be an egg donation to the surrogate—in other words, even if the surrogate is using her own eggs, the law acts as if eggs were donated to her and her husband then does not consent to the donation, so his rights are eliminated)

(All other states do not specifically address surrogacy.)

Surrogacy is an emotional issue for many people, which is why the states do not agree. Some people vehemently oppose it, suggesting it is like selling a baby or renting a womb. Other people feel it is a logical extension of adoption and is an option that presents couples with a greater opportunity to bond with the baby and include the birth mother in the child's life.

The Legal Process of Surrogacy

In states that do not have laws stating otherwise, when a woman gives birth to a child, she is the legal mother of the child, even if she is not the biological mother of the child or has entered into a surrogacy contract. If the woman is married, her husband is considered to be the child's legal father.

When a surrogacy agreement is entered into, the surrogate's husband must be a party to the contract and must revoke his rights to the child. If the intended father is the biological father, he can obtain an *order of paternity* (in some states this can happen during the pregnancy). This gives him the legal right to have access to the child at the hospital and to take the child home without any additional legal steps. The next step that must happen is that the intended mother must adopt the child in a second-parent adoption procedure. (See Chapter 17 for more information.) A few states that do not require stepparent adoption by the intended mother include Arkansas, Florida, and West Virginia (adoption is not required if the intended parents provided the embryo).

California Procedure

California is one of the few states that has a fairly well-established procedure for legalizing a surrogate birth. The intended parents file a court case during the pregnancy. The surrogate and her husband consent to the surrogacy in the case. The court issues a judgment that the intended parents are the legal parents. The intended parents then can inform the hospital of this and the birth certificate will be issued to them. They have the right to select the child's name.

However, if the surrogate provides the egg, she cannot relinquish her rights until the child is born (as in an adoption proceeding). In this case, the intended father can bring a paternity case during the pregnancy. Then the surrogate and her husband consent and the intended father is the legal father. The intended mother must use the second-parent adoption procedure to legalize her role.

Surrogacy Programs

Many couples locate a surrogate through a surrogacy program managed through a fertility clinic. Adoption agencies also often coordinate surrogacy programs. These programs locate potential surrogates, prescreen them, and match them with parents.

The ideal surrogate is married and has children of her own—this is because she is presumed to be mature and in a stable relationship. Being married means she has support from her husband and also has someone to financially support her during pregnancy. It also means that, presumably, most of her emotional needs are being met and she will not look to the baby to fulfill them. Having children is important because it means she understands what it is like to be pregnant and give birth. It is supposedly easier for her to carry this child for someone else and walk away if she has a real understanding of what pregnancy and birth are like and really knows the kinds of emotions she may feel after giving birth.

A woman who has never had children may be surprised at how strongly she feels about the baby when it is born and may be unable to give it up. The thinking is that a surrogate who is a parent has been through it all and enters the agreement with experience. This does not mean that a married surrogate with children of her own will not change her mind—but it does tend to improve the odds. Adoption agencies that have surrogacy programs treat the entire process in the same way they would a regular adoption and require home studies, counseling, and communication between the parties.

It is important to choose a surrogacy program that you feel comfortable with and confident in. Once you find a potential surrogate, it is necessary that she undergo physical and mental exams before any contract is entered into. The surrogate will also want to get to know you and decide if she feels comfortable with you. You, of course, will do the same with her. Since surrogacy involves a large degree of trust, it is important to use a surrogate you are completely comfortable with.

Finding a Surrogate on Your Own

Another option for surrogacy is to locate a surrogate on your own, without using a program. A sister, relative, or close friend may be willing to be a surrogate. Of course, in this situation, it is essential to use a reproductive law attorney who will advise you as to the laws in your state and will draw up a contract. Additionally, it is important that everyone involved in the surrogacy process obtain counseling, since this emotional situation is further compounded by the existing relationships. It is possible to locate a stranger surrogate on your own, but this is not recommended since you cannot perform the same sophisticated screening and psychological evaluation an agency or clinic can.

Surrogacy Agreements

Surrogacy agreements are complicated and important documents. The most important feature of a surrogacy agreement is that it revokes all rights and responsibilities the surrogate and her husband have to the child. The intended parents are the legal parents to the child. Other important clauses include:

- the surrogate agrees to follow all medical advice, but medical decisions during the pregnancy are ultimately left up to her;
- the surrogate agrees to consider selective reduction if necessary;
- the state where the child will be born is specified;
- the intended parents take on all financial and medical responsibility for the child;
- the intended parents have the right to name the child;
- the surrogate agrees to use her own medical insurance if she has any to cover her care during the pregnancy and delivery; and,
- the surrogate agrees to abstain from intercourse for a period of time while conception is attempted.

It is essential that you use an attorney experienced in surrogacy agreements. Even if you are working with an agency or surrogacy program, you should hire your own attorney to review the contract.

> **From the Expert**
>
> Read a sample surrogacy contract at:
> **www.surrogacy.com/legals/ gestcontract.html**
> **www.surromomsonline.com/ articles/contract.htm**
> **www.everything surrogacy.com/ cgi-bin/main.cgi?test**

Some people may wonder why an agreement is so essential, particularly if they live in a state where the courts will not uphold a surrogacy agreement. Even if your courts will not enforce a surrogacy agreement, it would still be important evidence should you get into a custody battle with your surrogate. Agreements are also important because the negotiation process can help you spot and work out things that might be potential problems down the line. The agreement will spell out in clear terms what everyone is going to do and how all the issues involved will be handled. Also, when people sign their name to a contract, they will usually feel obligated to carry out what they are agreeing to, so the agreement is an important way for both you and the surrogate to commit to the surrogacy.

Payment Issues

The issue of paying surrogates is probably the most controversial part of the entire surrogacy process. Some people argue that paying a surrogate amounts to buying a baby and should be outlawed. Others feel that surrogates should be compensated for their time, physical discomfort, emotional turmoil, and extreme generosity.

The intended parents will always take on all medical expenses relating to the conception, pregnancy, and birth. In many cases, you will also be permitted to reimburse the surrogate for travel expenses, maternity clothes, loss of wages, and additional child care expenses. The laws governing this are the same as the laws governing reimbursement of expenses for a birth mother in an adoption. (See Chapter 16 for more information.) Payment is often made through your attorney so there is a clear record that can be presented to the court as proof that all is done in a very forthright and honest manner.

Some states do permit payments to the surrogate to compensate her for time and discomfort. While payments are not permitted in other states, it is possible to give the surrogate a gift. Discuss this option with your attorney to find out what is permissible in your state. There may be rules about the value of the gift — it must really be a gift, not a form of payment. Some parents give their surrogate a special piece of jewelry or something else that has sentimental value and meaning. If you violate the law about payments, your parent-child relationship is not jeopardized, however, you may be subject to criminal penalties.

Insurance Coverage

If your surrogate has insurance coverage, it should cover her pregnancy. Some surrogates do not wish to use their own insurance. Others are willing to do so, if the intended parents pay all deductibles and co-pays. This is an important part of your agreement and should be included in your contract.

If your surrogate does not have health insurance coverage or will not be using her own coverage, you will need to pay for her medical expenses yourself or help her obtain a health insurance policy (which may mean paying for it yourself). Your insurance will not provide coverage until the birth, and then only if one parent is already a legal parent or if the child is officially placed with you as part of the adoption process.

Problems with Surrogacy

Many people are leery of surrogacy agreements, having heard about high-profile cases in which surrogates changed their minds and refused to place the child with the intended parents. In some ways, the prospect of this is scarier than that of an adoption in which the birth mother changes her mind, since in most cases, the intended father is also the biological and legal father of the baby.

Perhaps the most famous case about surrogacy is the *Baby M* case from New Jersey in 1988. In that case, the court invalidated the surrogacy agreement, but placed the baby with the biological father. The intended mother was not permitted to adopt since the surrogate (who was the biological mother) did not give her consent. The court found that the surrogacy agreement was invalid because the surrogate was paid. If the agreement did not include payment, it would have been valid.

Another landmark case is the *Johnson v. Calvert* case decided in California in 1993. In this case, the surrogate was implanted with a zygote that was created using genetic material from both the intended mother and intended father. The surrogate was not biologically related to the child. The court held that the legal parents are those who were intended to be the parents under the agreement. According to the court, the parent of a surrogate child is whoever is intended by the parties to be the parent, not who is biologically related to the child or who carries the pregnancy.

An Ohio case, *Belsito v. Clark*, from 1994, held that unless legal waiver or consent is provided, the people who provide the genetic material for the child are the natural parents of the child. This means that if the surrogate provides the egg, she is the legal mother, but can give her consent for the adoption.

In most cases, a surrogate does not change her mind, especially when you use a respected surrogacy program that will carefully screen all potential surrogates and help you find a good match. However, should something go wrong and the surrogate changes her mind, you first need to consult an attorney so that you can fully understand the laws in your state. As described earlier in this chapter, some states will not enforce surrogacy contracts.

If the intended father is the biological father of the child, at the very minimum, he will have access to the child until the case is resolved. There is a very good chance that the father will be able to obtain custody, and through him, the intended mother would be able to have time with the child. If the surrogate provided the egg, she will at the very least be entitled to have contact with the child (unless the birth is in a state where surrogacy contracts are enforced). If the surrogate did not provide the egg, the case for the intended parents is stronger, but not completely decided unless your state enforces surrogacy agreements.

NOTE: *Some people go to California to enter into surrogacy contracts since the laws there are the clearest and have a definite legal procedure in place.*

The surrogate's husband would have an initial claim to the child, since any child born to a woman during marriage is legally considered to be her husband's legal child. However, DNA tests would make it clear who the real father is and the husband's claim would be denied.

If a surrogate is related to the child and she changes her mind, and your state does not uphold agreements, you are facing a situation where the child would have to split his or her time between you and the surrogate. It is for this reason that many people are particular about the states in which they enter into surrogacy agreements.

Other Steps to Protect Yourself

As soon as you have entered into a surrogacy agreement, it is essential that you have a will drawn up or update an existing will. You will want to name a *guardian* for your child should anything happen to you. You want to have a clear legal plan for who would care for your child should you and your spouse pass away.

If you must go through a second-parent adoption process to make the intended mother the legal mother, there will likely be weeks or months until the adoption is final. In this time period, the father will have all the legal rights to make medical decisions for the child, but the intended mother will only have these rights if they are given to her in writing. The father should execute a written consent giving the mother the right to make medical decisions for the child.

Choosing a Surrogacy Program Questionnaire

Name of Agency_____

Name of Contact Person_____

Date of Interview_____

Questions:

❏ How do you recruit and locate surrogates?_____
_____

❏ How do you screen potential surrogates?_____
_____

❏ How do you screen the intended parents?_____
_____

❏ Do you provide counseling for both surrogate and intended parents?
_____

❏ What is your role in coordinating the surrogacy?_____
_____

❏ What fees are involved?_____
_____

❏ Are the fees refundable if the surrogacy is not completed?_____
_____

❏ Does this differ with miscarriage as opposed to a surrogate who changes her mind?_____
_____

❏ Is there a waiting list?_____
_____

❏ How many potential surrogates do you have in the program?_____
_____

❏ How many intended parents are you working with now?_____
_____

❏ Will you work with surrogates brought in by the intended parents?__
_____

(continued)

❑ What kind of relationship do you recommend that intended parents have with their surrogate?_____

❑ Is there any postbirth contact with your program?_____

❑ Have any of your surrogates changed their minds after becoming pregnant?_____

❑ How do you handle this situation?_____

❑ How many births does your program have a year?_____

❑ How many total births have you had?_____

❑ How long have you been doing this?_____

❑ Can you provide the names of parents to contact for references?_____

❑ Do intended parents have the right to refuse proposed surrogates?____

❑ Does the surrogate have her own attorney when signing the agreement?

❑ What kind of background information do you provide about the surrogate?_____

❑ How do you deal with the surrogate's expenses?_____

❑ How are they accounted and paid for?_____

Chapter 10

Emerging Technologies

The technology of ART is always advancing and changing. There are new treatments and options on the horizon that may someday be widely available.

Nuclear Transfer

Nuclear transfer is a process in which the *nucleus* of an egg cell, the part that contains the genetic material, is removed and replaced with another nucleus. This procedure could be used by women who are unable to produce viable egg cells on their own. The intended mother's genetic material would be implanted into an egg donated by another woman. The egg would then carry the intended mother's genes, but would also contain *mitochrondrial genes* from the donor. These genes do not determine physical traits but can carry inherited diseases, so the resulting child would be influenced by the donor but would be directly related to the intended mother. This newly formed egg could then be inseminated and placed in the intended mother's uterus or in that of a surrogate. The procedure has been attempted with human eggs, but there have been no reported positive results at the time this book was written.

Another option with this technique would be to replace the nucleus of the donor egg with the nucleus from a sperm. The newly created egg would then be fertilized by a different sperm. A child born by this technique would have two genetic parents who are both male. Although this has not been attempted yet, it is something that would be of great interest to the gay community.

If this procedure ever does become available, it will be important to obtain complete consent of all the parties involved, including the woman who provides the donor egg. A complete medical history will be essential since the donor egg can carry disease. Additionally, it will be important that the contract completely revokes the donor's rights and responsibilities towards the egg and any resulting child. This procedure is currently banned in California under its human cloning law.

In Vitro Maturation

Instead of stimulating women's ovaries to produce mature eggs, this technique allows eggs to be matured in vitro in the laboratory. This technique can be used by women who will be using their own eggs, as well as donor eggs. Legal issues may include storage, record keeping, and donor issues with any donated material.

> **From the Expert**
>
> For more information on in vitro maturation, see:
> **www.infertilitytutorials.com/ procedures_members/ invitro.cfm**

Cytoplasmic Transfer

Some women produce eggs that have defective *cytoplasm*, the material that fills the egg and gives it energy. This technique removes cytoplasm from a donor egg and injects it into the mother's egg. At least thirty children have been born using this technique.

As with other egg donation procedures, it is important to obtain the consent of all the parties involved and to have a contract that completely removes the donor's rights and responsibilities towards the egg, the cytoplasm, and any child that is created from it.

This procedure has now been banned in the US. Any procedure involving the transfer of genetic materials without the fusion of egg and sperm now requires the oversight and involvement of the Food and Drug Administration (FDA). The FDA has said they will require testing before they will approve the procedure. It is still possible to have this procedure performed in other countries, and some US couples have traveled overseas to use this technology. Taiwan, Israel, and Lebanon perform these procedures along with other countries.

> **From the Expert**
>
> For more information on cytoplasmic transfer, go to: **www.inciid.org/article.php? cat=infertility101&id=323**

Additionally in the United Kingdom, there is at least one physician that is using a cytoplasmic transfer technique using the intended mother's own eggs and cytoplasm and not using anything from a donor.

Cloning

Cloning is the most controversial area of ART and has received a lot of media coverage in the past few years. The type of cloning used in reproduction is called *somatic nuclear cloning* and is the same type that was used to create Dolly the sheep.

There are numerous applications of cloning that are useful in ART and too often they are obscured by the emotional reaction people have to the word *cloning*. Most people think of cloning as the process by which an exact replica of a specific human is created. With that technique, the nucleus of an embryo is removed and is replaced with DNA from an adult. It is then implanted. The result is an exact genetic twin to the person who donated the DNA.

Other applications may prove more useful and less controversial. Both sperm and eggs can be cloned, so a couple seeking ART could go through just one ART egg harvesting cycle, clone the harvested eggs, and then have innumerable eggs available for future fertilization. This would avoid the need to go through *superovulation* and the discomfort of the egg harvesting procedure again. Additionally, if a man has a low sperm count, his sperm could be cloned, making it possible to attempt many more insemination procedures.

From the Expert

Clonaid, a human cloning company, has reported the birth of five babies through the use of cloning. For more information about this company, see:

www.clonaid.com

Another type of cloning is *embryo cloning*. An infertile couple could create just one successfully fertilized embryo and clone it so numerous attempts at implantation could be made.

It should also be noted that there are other types of cloning used by medical science that do not involve the reproduction of humans. These other types of cloning are used to find cures for various diseases and for scientific research. They do not involve the creation of an identical human being or even a human embryo.

NOTE: *Clonaid is run by a religious cult called the Raelians. If you want more information about news reports about this group, do an Internet search using their name. The group is controversial and they have not yet provided any proof of their cloning claims.*

Legal Prevention

There has been much talk about passing laws to prevent cloning. Currently only a few states have created legislation banning reproductive cloning, including: Arkansas, California, Iowa, Michigan, North Dakota, Rhode Island, and Virginia. Louisiana had a law prohibiting reproductive cloning, but at the time this book was printed, the law had expired and had not yet been renewed.

Choosing Cloning

While reproductive cloning is not readily available, it is an option that may become more viable in the future. Should you ever consider cloning, it will be important to distinguish between the types of reproductive cloning being offered to you. Since little data is available about the long-term effect of human reproductive cloning, it will be a good idea to review the results of studies that have been conducted and to evaluate all long-term data available. Additionally, it will be important to ensure that the laboratory and facilities performing the procedure are experienced and have had past successes with the treatment being sought—the number of take home babies per procedures performed.

> **From the Expert**
>
> For more information about human cloning, see the new *Human Clone Rights Foundation* website (coming soon):
> **www.humanclonerights.org**

Carefully read all contracts and have them closely reviewed by a reproductive law attorney before signing anything. It will be important to understand what procedures are in place to label and identify genetic material that is being stored and worked on; what medical procedures will be used to create the pregnancy; and, all the costs and fees involved in the procedure.

Many people have moral and religious views about cloning as a reproductive choice, thus it is important to completely understand what genetic material is being duplicated; what the resulting child will be like; and, how all of these facts impact the parents.

Legal Ramifications of Cloning

There are few legal ramifications to cloning egg or sperm cells, if they are for one's own use. If cells such as these are cloned and then donated, the issues involved are similar to those for other sperm or egg donations, except children resulting from multiple cloned eggs or sperms would be more genetically similar than is usual in egg or sperm donation situations.

Embryo cloning creates embryos that are identical multiples. Couples using this technology might have identical twins born at the same time or could have one child and later have another child from a cloned embryo, creating genetic twins that are born years apart. Although identical twins have the same DNA, there are differences between them that stem from their environment. Children created using this method would have identical DNA and thus could not be distinguished using DNA tests. Other identifying features (such as scars or growth differences) can be used to distinguish them, should it ever be necessary. Modern fingerprinting is also able to discern the difference between identical twins most of the time.

Somatic nuclear cloning of an adult raises legal issues similar to that of embryo cloning. The child that is born would have DNA identical to the parent's, making him or her an identical twin to the parent. However, as with embryo cloning, environment would have an impact on the child and thus, he or she could not be exactly the same as the parent and it would be possible to distinguish between them.

Chapter 11

Cryopreservation

Cryopreservation, the subzero freezing of human cells, has opened many doors and provided a lot of flexibility for ART. Cryopreservation is used to freeze sperm, eggs (although this application is not completely foolproof yet), and embryos and save them for future use by the person or couple who created them or save them for donation to other infertile singles or couples. Cryopreservation is an important option for those facing chemotherapy, which can permanently damage sperm and egg production capabilities, or for women who are approaching menopause and may not be able to produce viable eggs in the future. Couples undergoing ART often choose to cryopreserve sperm, eggs, ovarian tissue, or embryos for later use. It is also possible to preserve eggs or sperm for use after your death.

Contract

The cryopreservation agreement is usually part of your overall contract with the clinic when you choose to undergo ART. When you choose to cryopreserve your reproductive material, make sure your contract addresses:

- cost;
- ownership (and addresses issues such as death or divorce);
- length of preservation;
- disposal or donation preferences;
- cryopreservation technique;
- steps that have been taken by the facility to protect the frozen material in a disaster, such as loss of power;

- what will happen if the facility closes (whether you will be given notice and time to transfer your material to another facility); and,
- the success rate with material that has been cryopreserved at that facility.

When you receive donated sperm, eggs, or embryos, you may have the option of cryopreserving the material you do not use immediately. Should you choose to do so, make sure your contract includes the items mentioned above, as well as:
- relinquishment of rights by donor(s);
- agreement that the genetic material can be used or frozen for future use;
- disclosure of genetic risk factors and family medical history by the donor;
- waiver of any right to collect child support against the donor(s); and,
- identification of recipient(s) as legal parent(s).

Cost
There is usually an upfront fee for cryopreservation (up to $1000) and then a monthly storage fee. Any fees for IVF, insemination, or embryo transfer would be completely separate and not included in this fee.

Divorce
There have been several high-profile cases about disputes among divorced couples about how their cryopreserved eggs, sperm, and embryos are to be used.

In New Jersey, in *J.B. v. M.B.* (June 2000), the court determined that frozen embryos from the marriage could be destroyed even though only one party agreed. In New York, *Maureen Kass v. Stephen Kass* (May 1998) held that even though the ex-wife wanted to implant the embryos, the embryos should be donated for research as the couple had agreed at the time they entered treatment.

There is a general consensus emerging among courts that there is a right *not* to be a parent. The position is that taking someone's genetic material and using it to create a child they do not want is almost a kind of rape and a violation of basic human rights. The issue is inflammatory because it again comes down to basic differences about how embryos should be treated and what legal status they should be given. Many clinics now include a clause in the contract stating that both the husband and wife must consent to the use, donation, or destruction of cryopreserved embryos.

Some states are beginning to address this situation. For example, in Florida, a written agreement is required that deals with what will happen with the eggs, sperm, or embryos in the event of a divorce.

It is a very good idea to designate in your cryopreservation agreement exactly what is to happen to the embryos in the event of divorce or death of one or both partners. The *Kass* decision in New York stated that the court should always look to the original agreement and try to uphold it no matter what changes happen in the meantime. This means that when you are making these decisions, you should carefully think through the various scenarios that could confront you in the future and how you would want the embryos to be handled in those situations.

Death of a Parent

Another troublesome issue has been the use of cryopreserved eggs, sperm, or embryos after the death of one of the intended parents. Some parents have had difficulty having their child legally recognized as the child of the predeceased parent. Some states have stepped in to legislate this issue with all of the following recognizing the deceased's parentage:

- Colorado
- Florida
- Louisiana
- North Dakota
- Texas
- Virginia
- Washington
- Wyoming

A Massachusetts case, *Woodward v. Commissioner of Social Security* (January 2002), held that children born to a parent after his or her death can inherit from him or her under the state's inheritance laws.

If you have cryopreserved material or if you plan to cryopreserve material, it is important to include information about it in your will. It is possible to pass ownership of this material to your spouse, your children, or anyone else you choose. It is important to think about these issues now and decide how you would want the genetic material handled so that you can be sure your wishes will be carried out.

Chapter 12

Raising an ART Child

Raising a child conceived with ART is like raising any other child, except you have some additional challenges. You must decide how and when you will explain your child's conception to him or her. You also must deal with reactions from others who learn of the path you took. Additionally, you will have to make choices about what, if any, contact your child will have now or in the future with donors or surrogates and deal with any possible health consequences your child will face.

Explaining Things to Your Child

Some parents never tell their child that they used ART to achieve conception, while others feel an obligation to explain this to the child. The path you take is your choice. Parents who use ART, but do so without a donor or surrogate, may feel there is no need to explain the complicated procedures to a child and may save the explanation for when the child is older.

If you do feel that you want to be open with your child, there are a number of things to consider.

- Do you want to share all the information you have about a donor or surrogate with your child?
- Do you want to paint this person in the same way you might a biological parent who placed a child for adoption?
- Is this donor or surrogate in more of a helper role in your mind?

Whatever explanation you choose can be challenging. Remember to only tell your child what he or she can handle at his or her current age. There are details children are not able to understand. Break it down into easy-to-understand explanations.

Coping with Other People

While your close friends and family may be aware of your use of ART, they may not completely understand how you want to approach the topic and deal with it as you raise your child. If possible, it is best to set basic ground rules. You might want to be the only person who discusses this topic with your child, and may ask others not to mention it. If you have no plans to tell your child, then you will need to be sure friends and family can keep a secret. If you have a specific approach you want to take in explaining the ART circumstances to your child, be sure to tell your family and friends how you are going to approach this.

As your child grows, there will be other circumstances when the information about his or her conception will become relevant. Your pediatrician will need to know all the information about the conception of your child and the medical history of donors or surrogates may become important at some point should your child develop certain illnesses or conditions. Your child may bring up his or her conception at school or with friends and you may be required to step in and give more accurate explanations.

From the Expert

See Appendix A for additional books about assisted reproduction. Some books about assisted reproduction are available at:

www.donor-conception-network.org/basechild books.htm

You may have various uncomfortable encounters where people will assume your child is genetically related to you or your spouse, when in fact he or she is not. Some parents choose to ignore these comments or gloss over them since they feel no need to explain their family's intimate details. Other parents feel a need to set the record straight.

If you are a single parent or a gay couple, people may ask uncomfortable questions about your child's biological parentage. Again, different parents have different reactions to these comments. You will have to find the path with which you are most comfortable.

Medical Information

If you use a donor or surrogate, you will receive medical history information. It will be important to save this information for your child. If the clinic or sperm bank you work with updates donors' medical information, ask if you will automatically receive updates when they are available or if you will have to contact the clinic or bank to obtain updated information.

Helping Your Child Locate His or Her Donors or Surrogates

When your child is a teen or an adult, he or she may wish to find and meet the donor or surrogate who participated in his or her conception. Some sperm banks will receive requests from children and forward them to donors, while others will not. If this opportunity is something you want to make available to your child, make sure to ask the bank's policy about this before selecting a donor. Some egg donor clinics are willing to pass along requests from children as well, but since egg donors are less common than sperm donors, this does not happen as frequently. There is generally no contact information available about embryo donation, unless it is handled similar to an open adoption.

Other sperm banks allow children or parents to make contact with other families that used the same donor's sperm, allowing the children to meet and have relationships with their half siblings.

From the Expert

ART children and parents can try to locate donors using donor registries, such as this one:

www.abolishadoption.com/ DonorOffspring.html

Parents can try to locate their children's half-siblings through registries, such as this one:

http://mattes.home. pipeline.com/sibling.html

Chapter 13

Moving from Fertility to Adoption

You may reach a point where you decide you are finished pursuing your options with assisted reproduction and want to consider adoption. This is a personal decision and is one you must make yourself. Often this is not an easy choice or one that comes quickly.

Some couples choose to pursue fertility and adoption at the same time, believing that only one or the other will work, but are happy to be doubly blessed if both result in a child. You have the right to pursue both family-building options at the same time if you wish. Practically speaking, most couples usually only do one at a time since both adoption and fertility treatments are expensive and emotionally draining.

Some factors you may wish to consider when making the decision to pursue adoption are:

- The cost of the fertility treatments versus the cost of the type of adoption you would be interested in;
- The emotional and physical toll fertility treatments are creating on you and your spouse or partner;
- Your doctor's evaluation of your chances of success;
- Your financial situation;
- Your current situation — marital, career, health, age, and so on; and,
- The importance to you of having a biological link with your child.

The decision to move from fertility to adoption does not have to be a permanent decision. You could begin an adoption and then decide you really want to go back and try some other fertility procedures. There is no right answer and you can only do what seems right to you at the time.

The next section of this book discusses the different types of adoptions available. If you are considering adoption, read through it and educate yourself about the options that are available to you, as well as the costs and procedures involved. Getting some information may help you make a decision about where you want to go from here.

Section II

Adoption

Chapter 14

Understanding Adoption

Adoption is a way to create a family outside of biological means. Children who are adopted are children of their families just as much as biological children. In recent years, adoption has become less of a secret and more of a celebrated route to parenthood. If you are considering adoption, it is important to first understand some of the general rules.

Legal Effects

When a child is adopted, the birth parents' legal ties to the child are completely severed. The child no longer has any legal connection to these parents. The adoptive parents become the child's legal parents. A new birth certificate is issued with their names listed as the parents. An adopted child has the exact same rights as a couple's biological child. Adopted children have the right to:

- inherit from their adoptive parent(s) and adoptive families;
- take their parents' last name(s);
- collect benefits (such as Social Security) through their parent(s); and,
- rely on their parent(s) for support.

Additionally, should a child's adoptive parents ever divorce, custody and visitation will be decided in the same way as it would for biological children. Being adopted has no impact on custody and visitation since an adopted child is legally no different than a child that is born to a couple.

Even if the child is the biological child of one parent and is then adopted by the other parent, both parents have the same rights.

Birth Parents' Rights and Roles

When a child is born to a woman, she is legally the child's mother, unless and until a court issues an order stating otherwise. Birth fathers' rights are a little more slippery, simply because the identity of a child's biological father is not always obvious. If a woman is married when she gives birth, her husband is the legal father of the child, unless it is proven otherwise. If a woman is unmarried, a man can admit to being the father (by signing documents such as an *admission of paternity* or through what is called the *putative father registry*) or a court can issue an order determining paternity based on DNA testing.

When a child is adopted, both birth parents must *consent* to the adoption (unless the birth father is unknown or cannot be located). The adoption process affords both birth parents a period of time to change their minds about the adoption once the process is in motion. (See Chapter 16 for more information.)

Once the adoption process is finalized, the birth parents have no further legal rights to the child. They can never come back and decide they have changed their minds and want custody, and they do not have any right to see or spend time with the child. There are cases where birth parents later challenge an adoption, but this is not the norm and only occurs when there is some kind of abnormality or problem in the way the adoption process was handled (for example, if one of the birth parents was not properly notified). It is important to understand that in most states, the birth parents have a period of time after the birth during which they can reconsider their consent to the adoption. This is not overturning the adoption; the adoption simply is not legal until this time period has ended.

Extended Birth Family

Adoption also severs the child's legal ties to the birth parents' families—grandparents, aunts, uncles, cousins, and so on. The child is no longer legally related to these people, which means these people have no claim to visitation with the child. There are also no longer any inheritance rights. For example, if a grandmother leaves everything to be divided equally among her grandchildren, a child who was placed for adoption with another family no longer qualifies as one of her grandchildren.

It is important to understand that adoption severs not only the rights of the birth family, but also their connection to the child. An adoption takes a child out of one family unit and places him or her into another. It is a complete and absolute substitution.

In some instances, however, a birth family continues to have contact with the child. It is becoming more common for a child to continue to have contact not only with birth parents, but also birth families. Despite the adoption, these people are a part of a child's history and even though the law changes their legal relationship, it is possible for them to continue to know each other. Often this is considered the healthiest way for an adoption to happen. You can change what a birth certificate says, but you cannot change a child's feelings. Continuing these family bonds can be important for older children who are adopted. This has to be done the right way, with the proper safeguards, so the child is not confused. (See Chapter 24 for more information.)

Legal Process

It is important to remember that the legal process is separate from the process you will go through to find a child to adopt. Finding a child can take much longer and can involve choosing an agency, finding a birth mother on your own, or dealing with the requirements of the foreign country your child will come from. (See Chapter 18 for information about agencies; Chapter 20 about independent adoptions; and, Chapter 19 about international adoptions.)

The *legal process* for adoption follows the same general path whether your adoption is a single-parent adoption, second-parent adoption, agency adoption, private adoption, or international adoption. The major components of the process include:

- a background check, where prospective parents are fingerprinted and have their backgrounds checked for criminal records;
- a home study, in which a social worker meets with the prospective parents and sees their home;
- the birth parents' consent to the adoption; and,
- the actual court procedure in which documents are submitted and reviewed, and the adoption is approved.

The legal process itself can take six months to a year. (See Chapter 16 for more information about the specific legal processes involved in adoption.)

Making the Decision to Adopt

If you are considering adopting through an agency, internationally, or directly through a private birth mother, consider joining an adoption support group. (See Appendix A for more information.) These groups can provide practical information, contact information, support, and advice. Talking to other parents who have adopted or who are going through the adoption process will provide you with a clear perspective on how the process works and how it affects parents.

A support group is an excellent way to make connections, get information, hear other people's experiences, and consider new approaches. For example, you might only be considering an agency adoption, but through a support group you might learn of a birth mother interested in independent adoption. You will meet other couples seeking to adopt, as well as families that have successfully adopted. You may also meet attorneys and other adoption professionals who can assist you with your adoption journey.

If you are considering a second-parent adoption, the decision process is a bit different since the child is already in your life. You are now confronting a legal decision, not a family-forming decision. This is a decision you must make with your partner or spouse and often with the child's input as well. Second-parent adoptions must also consider the child's other parent, if he or she is alive, since his or her consent will be necessary.

> **From the Expert**
> Locate an adoption group in your area using this resource: **www.stateadoptions.com**

Some people come to the adoption process after unsuccessfully attempting to conceive a child themselves, with or without assisted reproduction treatments. Others simply know that adoption is the way for them to create or add to a family. No matter what your reasons are, be sure they make sense to you and work for your family. Choosing between adopting and using infertility treatments can be a difficult one. Help weighing out your options and making a decision can be found in Chapter 13.

It is possible, and perfectly acceptable, to pursue adoption while undergoing infertility treatment, also called assisted reproductive treatment, such as IVF, GIFT, and other procedures. (See Chapter 1 for more information about these options.) An adoption agency will not turn you away, but it may make them think twice about whether you would choose not to complete the adoption should you become pregnant. Many couples feel that adoption and assisted reproduction is an either-or proposition, when in fact many couples do explore and pursue both choices simultaneously. Because both processes can be long, it may make sense to consider both.

> **From the Expert**
> If you are considering adoption, take an adoption self-assessment to help you and your partner (if any) get a clear sense as to how you feel about the many choices available. One is available at:
> **http://adoption.about. com/library/adopt/ blselfeval.htm**

Preparing for the Adoption Rollercoaster

No matter what kind of adoption you are considering or have selected, it is likely that the process will be emotional. Choosing to create a family is one of the most private decisions, yet when you choose to do so through adoption, suddenly there are social workers; lawyers; adoption case managers; and judges scrutinizing you, your life, your decision, your abilities, and your desirability. It can be disconcerting and frustrating to know that the future of your family is in large part in the hands of these strangers. It also can be frustrating to realize that people who have biological children can have them without any approval or screening (and sometimes with little thought), but someone who desperately wants a child and wishes to adopt must go through an intrusive process.

Some adoption processes take longer and can be more difficult than others. If you are hoping to adopt a newborn in the United States, you may realize that finding a birth mother is a long and difficult process. If you are planning a second-parent adoption, you might be frustrated by the hoops that must be jumped through to make legal something that seems and feels obvious to you.

While waiting to adopt, it is important to have patience. Do everything you can to make the paperwork go smoothly. Never lose your belief that you will find your child.

While none of the adoption processes are as simple as sperm meeting egg, they are not as scary and drawn out as some people expect. Remember that the reward at the end is a child. That will make everything feel worthwhile.

Preparing for the Future

When you decide to adopt, your decision affects not only you and your partner, if you have one, but also your entire extended family. It also, of course, affects the child you bring into your family. Adoption is a decision that you may make today, but will impact the long-term future in many ways. When making the decision, it is important to consider how it will affect you and your family in the long term.

You must also give some thought to how your decision will affect the child you adopt. The type of adoption you choose will have an impact on your child. If you use an agency adoption, your child will probably grow up with little or no contact with his or her birth parents. If you use independent adoption, it is likely your child will have some sort of contact with, or at least will know how to contact, his or her birth parents. International adoption usually completely rules out any hope of your child having any contact with the birth parents. The results of any of these paths can have a long-term impact on you and your child, so it is important to consider every angle as you are making your decision.

Chapter 15

Adoption Decisions

Once you have chosen to adopt, you will find that there are many more decisions ahead of you. You must choose:
- the type of adoption you are interested in;
- the people who will help you; and,
- what kind of relationship you want to have with the birth parents in the future.

Open vs. Closed Adoption

Adoptions used to be done in complete secrecy, with even the child being kept in the dark. Today, things have changed and most people are more honest about adoptions. Most adoptive children now grow up understanding that they were adopted. This concept of an *open adoption* is one in which the adoptive and birth parents have some contact (that can vary greatly) and the child knows that he or she is adopted. The child may even know or have contact with the birth parents.

The degree of contact can range from minimal to very involved. For example, some adoptive parents see the birth mother frequently during the pregnancy, attend the birth, and continue to see her and have contact with her throughout the child's life. In other situations, an open adoption can mean that the adoptive parents meet the birth mother once, learn her first name, and obtain copies of her family medical history. A middle-road alternative includes some meetings or contact during pregnancy and photos and letters exchanged occasionally throughout the child's life.

The type of adoption you pursue will affect how open it is to some degree. *International adoptions* provide no contact with birth parents; *private adoptions* can be some of the most open; and *domestic agency adoptions* can vary greatly depending on the agency's policies, your wishes, and the birth mother's wishes.

From the Expert

You can read sample open adoption agreements online at:

http://public.findlaw.com

Choosing an open or closed adoption depends on your personal feelings. It is important to understand that your adoption will not be specified as an open one or a closed one in your adoption papers. The court cannot require you to send photos to the birth mother, but it cannot prevent you from having a relationship with her either. As far as the court is concerned, the adoptive parents become the legal parents and the birth parents have no further rights once the adoption is completed. The adoption legal process completely ends the birth parents' legal rights, but anything you choose to do from that point is up to you. It is important to realize that some birth mothers will not agree to the adoption if they do not feel you have made a commitment to the level of openness (or closure) they are seeking.

An important consideration in open adoption is how very real the baby and birth mother can be to you as you are waiting for the birth. This can be wonderful, because in a way you are included in the pregnancy process. It can also be heartbreaking if the birth mother ultimately decides not to go through with the adoption. Because you are so heavily invested in the situation and because the baby and birth mother are so much a part of you life, it can be emotionally very difficult to cope if the adoption is not completed.

From the Expert

For more information about open adoption, contact the *American Association of Open Adoption Agencies* at:

www.openadoption.org

An open adoption can place more pressure on the adoptive parents. They must meet and be interviewed by the agency, by the social worker who does the home study, and sometimes by the birth mother. It can be very difficult to sit in a room with a woman who is carrying what might be your baby and try to measure up to whatever standards she is using.

Some adoptive parents find that the relationship they carry on with the birth mother during the pregnancy can be emotionally draining. Some people never feel quite sure how involved to get, what kind of help to offer, or even what to say at certain times. Your agency can help guide you through this process for the most part, but it is something to consider.

Finally, some adoptive parents simply do not want the specter of the birth mother intruding on their lives. They do not want to meet or interact with her or think too much about her role or her connection to the baby once that child becomes theirs. Many adoptive parents feel she will exert some kind of emotional influence over the child and always be the *real* mother. These are individual decisions you must make on your own. As always, an adoption support group can help you through these thought processes and decisions.

Domestic vs. International Adoption

Choosing between adopting a child within the United States or from another country is a common dilemma faced by potential adoptive parents. With domestic adoptions, it is generally easier to adopt a younger and possibly healthier child than it is to adopt from another country. However, international adoptions tend to be quicker and can be less costly.

The following two lists identify the pros and cons to each option. Choose the path that is most comfortable for you and your family.

> **From the Expert**
>
> Information to help you consider domestic versus international adoption is available at:
> **www.adoptall.com/ intguide.html**

Domestic Adoption

Pros:

- It is easier to adopt a newborn.
- The child is usually healthy and developmental delays are limited.
- You can obtain complete medical records for the baby.
- You can obtain complete family medical history.
- Everything is conducted in English.
- You may be able to meet or have contact with the birth parents.
- The agency you are working with may be the one the child is placed through (which can simplify things).
- As complicated as the adoption process is, it is done only using the laws of this country and the requirements are very clear.

Cons:

- These adoptions generally take a year or longer.
- You may have to wait longer to get a newborn.
- You may have to deal with a birth mother who could change her mind after the baby is born.
- Your child may be able to one day meet and know the birth parents.
- You may have to meet a birth mother's selection criteria.

International Adoption

Pros:

- These adoptions generally happen more quickly.
- There is no shortage of children available.
- The cost of the adoption is usually less than with domestic adoption.
- You gain not only a child but an entire culture that becomes part of your family.

Cons:

- The child you adopt is usually no younger than three or four months old (newborns are not available because of the way the process works).
- Children may not be in good health and may have developmental delays.
- You may get little or no medical information about your child or his or her family.
- You will have the added expense of travel.
- The red tape you may need to deal with in your child's country of origin may be extensive.

Agency vs. Private Adoption

An *agency adoption* is one in which you work with an agency that will locate a child for you to adopt and provides most, if not all, the related services. In a *private adoption*, you locate a birth mother on your own—through adoption attorneys, adoption facilitators, or on your own (often through word of mouth or by placing newspaper ads). However, many adoptive parents who

From the Expert

One of the most comprehensive and helpful resources available to parents seeking to adopt is the *National Adoption Information Clearinghouse*. Its website is almost certain to provide answers to almost any question you have. Find it at:

http://naic.acf.hhs.gov

do private adoptions use an agency to handle the adoption once the birth mother is located.

Some agencies can be difficult to work with, but when pursuing a private adoption, the entire process can be even more complicated. With each method having its own set of pros and cons, you must decide which one best suits your situation. Review the two lists on the following pages to help in your decision making.

Agency Adoption

Pros:

- The agency locates the child and does the legwork.
- The agency provides the social worker for the home study.
- The agency provides counseling and services.
- The agency is in charge of the adoption and moving it along.
- A good agency has plenty of children to adopt.
- The agency can help manage your relationship with the birth parents.
- The agency screens birth parents and usually chooses those less likely to change their minds.
- The search time may be shorter since the agency already has a network set up to locate birth mothers.
- The agency screens the adoptive parents and chooses those that the birth parents will not object to.

Cons:

- The agency is in charge and things move at their pace, not yours.
- The agency can screen you out if they feel you are not desirable.
- You have no actual control over the process.
- You must pay agency fees in addition to other adoption expenses.

Private Adoptions

Pros:

- You have control of the situation.
- You can develop the kind of relationship with the birth mother that feels right to you.
- You decide the pace at which the process moves.
- You can personally find and select a birth mother.
- You have more information about the birth parents.
- There are fewer people involved.
- There are no agency fees.
- You can immediately begin to bond with the child and can have extensive contact with the birth mother during the pregnancy.

Cons:

- The process can be riskier, with the birth mother more likely to change her mind.
- You may need to spend a lot of time searching or advertising for birth mothers.
- You do not have as many professionals guiding you and supporting you.
- You are responsible for understanding the laws of your state or finding an attorney to guide you as you look for birth mothers.
- The costs are more unpredictable.
- You cannot select the gender of the child—whatever your birth mother has, you get.
- It can be more stressful than going through an agency.

Finding and Choosing an Agency

If you choose to work with an agency to adopt, it will be important to take some time to interview several agencies and choose the one that you are most comfortable with and confident in. You will be paying the agency a lot of money and you want to make sure that you get the results you want.

If you are seeking to do an international adoption or a domestic adoption (which is not a private adoption or a second-parent adoption), you will have to use an agency. Agencies can be profit or nonprofit, but both still charge fees. Agencies may be public (run by the state) or private (run by a private company). Agencies can also be religious or nonsectarian, but it is important to know that most religious-based agencies do not require adoptive parents to be members of that religion.

An agency cannot reject you because of race or religion. However, marital status can be used as a determining factor, as can sexual orientation.

The best way to locate an agency is by word of mouth, through adoption support groups, or through people you know who have used an agency successfully. Once you have a few names of agencies to consider, make an initial phone call and request information by mail. If the agency has a website, be sure to visit it. Many agencies provide informational meetings you can attend to learn more about the agency as well as the adoption process. Do not sign up with any agency before you have time to ask questions, compare it to others, and think about the decision. Ask about informational meetings and be sure to attend them. Ask questions and be observant. If you still feel the agency is a possibility, schedule an interview and use the questionnaire beginning on page 115 to evaluate and record responses.

One thing you will need to get a clear picture of is the agency's fee. The agency will collect fees to cover the home study, application, birth mother's expenses (if it is a domestic adoption), and other costs. Some agencies will clearly enunciate these separate amounts for you. Be wary of an agency that lumps total costs together and will not provide a breakdown.

Call your state's agency that licenses and monitors adoption agencies (your social services or family and children department) and ask for information about the adoption agency, including its history and any complaints that have been filed against it. Ask to speak to an adoption specialist in the department and question the agency's reputation.

The average length of time for an adoption should be under two years. If an agency has a longer average, you may want to go somewhere else.

When you have chosen an agency, make sure you get everything in writing so there can be no confusion or dispute. You will need to sign a contract with the agency that will spell out the fees, procedures, and responsibilities. (See Chapters 18 and 19 for more information about evaluating agencies.)

Finding and Choosing an Attorney

No matter what type of adoption you choose to pursue, you will need an attorney to represent you. It is important to select an attorney who is experienced in handling adoptions. If you have an attorney you have used for other matters, ask him or her for a referral. Ask members of your adoption support group for referrals. You can also call your state or city bar association and ask for a referral.

Once you have some attorneys to consider, schedule a free consultation. Use the *Attorney Evaluation Questionnaire* at the end of the chapter to help you evaluate the attorney. Make sure you get a clear picture of the attorney's fees. If you are seeking a private adoption, you will need to find out if the attorney is able to help you locate birth mothers or if he or she will only handle the legal paperwork.

Expect attorney fees to range from $2000 to $7000, depending on the type of adoption and where you live. Avoid attorneys who seek *contingency fees* (paid only if they accomplish certain things such as finding a child for you to adopt). This can motivate an attorney to use nonethical means to find a child for you to adopt. Make sure that when you do select an attorney, that your agree-

> **From the Expert**
>
> For a referral to an attorney, contact:
> American Academy of
> Adoption Attorneys
> P.O. Box 33053
> Washington, DC 20033
> 202-832-2222
> **www.adoptionattorneys.org**

ment with him or her is in writing and is in the form of a retainer agreement or retainer letter.

Facilitators

Adoption *facilitators* are professionals who locate birth mothers for adoptive parents. They can play an ongoing role throughout the adoption process and take on a coordinating position similar to that an agency plays. Be aware that many states do not permit the use of adoption facilitators. Some states do permit facilitators to operate, but do not license or regulate them. (California does license facilitators.) Be sure to talk to your attorney about the legalities of using a facilitator. Also, be certain to check references and backgrounds of any facilitators you consider. Do not work with anyone without a contract and make sure that your attorney approves the contract.

The following states do not permit paid adoption facilitators:
- Colorado
- Florida
- Georgia
- Kentucky
- Maryland
- Missouri
- New Jersey
- New York
- Oklahoma
- Oregon
- Tennessee
- Virginia
- West Virginia

It is important to distinguish between paid and unpaid facilitators. Unpaid facilitators are the way many adoptions happen. A minister, doctor, therapist, or nurse might work with a woman who is pregnant and help her find an agency or an adoptive family. These facilitators are doing nothing wrong. Many states object to *paid* facilitators. Part of the problem is that these kinds of facilitators fall outside the specific requirements that states place on adoption agencies and can operate on their own. There may come a time when all states will license, regulate, and allow facilitators, but for now, you must be very clear about what your state permits and does not permit.

If you can use a facilitator, the advantage is that the relationship is more personal than with an agency. He or she personally (for the most part) handles the details of your adoption and is personally accountable to you. The downside is that in most states, a facilitator is not licensed or regulated and operates completely on his or her own, with no safeguards for adoptive families and no required training.

> **From the Expert**
>
> For more information on state laws about facilitators and other adoption laws, visit:
> **www.theadoptionguide.com**

Affording Adoption

When considering adoption, many people are taken aback by the costs involved. It can be particularly difficult to accept the costs if you are adopting a special needs child. However, affording adoption can be easier than you think. Once you have adopted a child, you are eligible for tax credit to reimburse you for expenses. (See Chapter 16 for more information.) Many employers offer adoption cost partial reimbursement programs.

You may also wish to consider purchasing *adoption insurance*. It will reimburse you for expenses if a planned adoption does not take place. Adoption insurance can be difficult to locate, but one source is MBO Insurance Brokers in

> **From the Expert**
>
> For more information about adoption insurance, contact:
> *National Adoption Foundation*
> 100 Mill Plain Road
> Danbury, CT 06811
> 203-791-3811
> **www.nafadopt.org/ default.asp**

Menlo Park, California (800-833-7337). You might also talk to an insurance broker in your area.

NOTE: *These types of insurance policies often only apply if you work with agencies or attorneys on the list approved by the insurance carrier.*

The National Adoption Foundation has $9 million in revolving loans available to adoptive parents. Some of these loans are unsecured loans, meaning you do not put up any security, such as a house, to guarantee the loan. They also offer home equity loans in which your home is used as security for the loan. The loans typically average $2500 and are financed through MBNA bank.

Adoption is expensive, but it is not completely out of reach for most families. If you are considering adoption, you may wish to create a separate bank account and start saving what you can to help pay for the costs. Look into the special adoption loans available or consider a home equity loan through your own bank. You might also consider letting family and friends know you are saving for adoption and ask for contributions to your fund instead of holiday or birthday gifts. (Any person can give up to $11,000 tax free per year to any other person as a gift.)

If you are planning to add a child to your family, you already know that the child will bring added expenses. The money you earn now will have to stretch further to accommodate a child's needs. You can make adoption affordable by beginning to act like parents now — take the money it would cost to raise a child each week or each month and set that aside to help pay for the adoption.

Another consideration is comparing adoption expenses with assisted reproduction treatment expenses. The cost of adopting a child may turn out to be a lot less than pursuing months of unsuccessful fertility treatments. This is a choice you must weigh on your own, since obviously money is not the only consideration when choosing how you will add a child to your family.

Agency Evaluation
Questionnaire

Name of Agency_____

Name of Contact Person_____

Date of Interview_____

Questions:

❏ Are you licensed in this state?_____

_____

❏ How long have you been in business?_____

_____

❏ Can you provide references?_____

_____

❏ Do you handle domestic or international adoptions?_____
    ❏ If both, which do you place more often?_____

    _____

❏ Can you place children from other states?_____

_____

❏ Do you have religious restrictions?_____

_____

❏ What other guidelines or restrictions do you have in place?

_____

_____

❏ What is your fee structure?_____

_____

    ❏ Can you provide a breakdown?_____
    ❏ When are the amounts due?_____
    ❏ What fees are not included in this?_____

_____

❏ What is the average length of time for one of your adoptions?

_____

❏ How many placements do you make per year?_____
    ❏ How many in the last year?_____

(continued)

❏ How many people are on your waiting list to adopt?_____

❏ Do you have infants available?_____

    ❏ What is the average age of the children placed through
    your agency?_____

❏ What portion of fees are refundable if the adoption does not occur?

_____

❏ Please explain your home study process._____

_____

    ❏ How long does it take?_____

_____

❏ Can you provide a list of approved social workers to use for the home
study?_____

❏ Will you assist with a private adoption?_____

    ❏ What fees would apply?_____

_____

❏ How are your birth mothers located?_____

_____

❏ Who makes the placement decision—the agency or the birth mother?

_____

    ❏ How is placement decided?_____

_____

❏ What is your position on open adoption?_____

_____

    ❏ What kind of relationship do you encourage or advise for birth
    parents and adoptive parents?_____

_____

❏ Do you provide counseling for birth and adoptive parents?_____

_____

    ❏ Are there additional fees for this?_____

    ❏ What is involved in the counseling process?_____

_____

❏ What medical history information is provided to adoptive parents about the birth parents?_____

   ❏ Are birth mothers screened for HIV and other conditions?_____

❏ If potential adoptive parents turn down a birth mother, may they continue in the program and receive the next available placement?_____

❏ If an adoption is not completed, can the expenses be transferred or rolled over to a new birth mother?_____

❏ What other services does the agency provide?_____

❏ What is your policy on divorce, singles, and families with biological children?_____

❏ Do you have a grievance policy?_____

   ❏ If so, how does it work?_____

   ❏ If not, how are problems resolved?_____

Attorney Evaluation
Questionnaire

Name of Firm_____

Name of Attorney_____

Date of Interview_____

Questions:

❑ How long have you practiced adoption law?_____
_____

❑ What states are you licensed in?_____
_____

❑ How many adoptions do you handle per year?_____
_____

❑ How many have you handled in the last six months?_____
_____

❑ Do you handle domestic or international adoptions or both?_____
_____

    ❑ What percent of your practice is made up of these two types?
_____

❑ Do you handle private adoptions?_____
_____

    ❑ How many have you handled?_____
_____

    ❑ What role do you take in the private adoption process?_____
_____

❑ What are your fees?_____
_____

    ❑ Do you charge a flat fee or an hourly rate?_____
_____

        ❑ What kind of payment schedule do you use?_____
_____

❑ Can you recommend any agencies that you have worked with in the past?_____
_____

❑ How long does the average adoption process take?_____
_____

Chapter 16

Adoption Procedures

While there are a variety of different types of adoption to consider and choose from, some things are common to all the choices. You will need a home study; you will need to understand the issues of consent and revocation of consent by birth parents; and, you will face a court procedure to finalize the adoption. This chapter provides an overview of these considerations and procedures. Later chapters will discuss specifics that apply to each different type of adoption.

Home Studies

A *home study* is an evaluation and investigation of prospective parents' histories, parenting abilities, home, lifestyle, and parenting abilities. Home studies are required in almost all adoptions, but in some states they may be waived for second-parent adoptions. (See Chapter 17 for more information.)

A home study is done by a licensed *social worker*. When working with an agency, the agency may have a list of social workers it works with or may have social workers who are employed by the agency. Make sure that the social worker you use is licensed in your state.

> **From the Expert**
> See a sample adoption home study online at:
> **www.1-800-home study.com/homestudy/ sample.html**

The home study is probably the most feared hurdle in the adoption process by many prospective parents. In reality, it is not nearly as terrifying as it may sound.

A social worker will come to your home, meet you and your spouse (if you have one), and ask you questions about your background. These questions can cover information such as:

- where you were born;
- your family;
- your education;
- your job history;
- any previous marriages;
- any previous addresses;
- any arrests or convictions; and,
- other children you have.

The social worker will also ask questions about your lifestyle and personal life. These questions can cover topics including:

- your employment schedule;
- income;
- friends and family you spend time with;
- organizations you belong to;
- pets;
- religious beliefs;
- hobbies and interests;
- smoking, drinking, and drug use;
- medical conditions;
- infertility and any treatments you have undergone or are undergoing;
- why you want to adopt;
- how you plan to make room in your life for a child;
- where the child will sleep;
- child care plans;
- how you will discipline a child; and,
- how you will adjust your finances to include a child.

There is no right answer to any of these questions. The most important thing you can do is be honest. Dishonesty is the biggest mistake you can make because it will usually be discovered and then the social worker and agency will have to wonder why you lied or what else you were not honest about.

In general, the purpose of the questions is to find out if you have a stable lifestyle, if you would be able to raise a child, if you have a support network in place (i.e., family and friends), if you are financially stable and can support a child, if your home is conducive to a child, and if you can emotionally handle being a parent. No parent is perfect, so no one is going to expect you to present a perfect picture of yourself.

You can prepare yourself for these questions by simply reading over the list of questions and thinking about what you might say. It is a mistake to prepare a script for yourself—to recite answers you have planned and memorized—but thinking through the questions in advance and coming up with some general ideas about how you will respond can make you feel more comfortable.

The social worker will want to see your home and will be particularly interested in where the child will sleep. Your home does not have to be spotless and it does not have to be childproof. However, it is a good idea to show that you understand the basics of childproofing and explain how you will make the home safe for a child.

You may need to meet with the social worker more than once to cover all the information that is needed. Do not become overwhelmed by this process. Some prospective parents spend weeks repainting the house and decorating a nursery. Doing so may make you seem a little overanxious, but it is certainly nothing the social worker has not seen before. Your home should simply be relatively clean and neat. This is not a contest to decide who would be the best parent. The home study is simply a way of making sure you are a decent person who is able to care for a child.

Additionally, you will be asked to write an autobiographical statement that will probably reiterate the information you provide verbally. This statement is brief—just a page or two—and should include information about why you want to adopt, as well as a brief history of your life. You will need to provide certified copies of birth and marriage certificates (as well as divorce decrees if applicable) and a medical report from your physician describing your health and explaining any conditions you have. You will also need written verification of your income (pay stubs or tax returns).

Another part of the home study is providing references—three to five people who know you well and can say nice things about you. This should include a variety of people, such as friends, neighbors, clergy, coworkers, and so on. They will be asked to provide letters explaining how they know you, how long they have known you, and why they believe you would make good adoptive parents.

Choose people who know you well. It would look strange to get a reference from someone who has only known you a short while. Select people that are themselves upstanding members of the community. It is always a good idea to include a reference from a minister, rabbi, or priest if you are involved in a church or temple. (It is okay if you are not religious and there is no need to join a church or temple just so you can get a letter of reference.)

In general, it is a good idea to choose people who have some kind of status—people with respected jobs, such as teachers, lawyers, business owners, and so on. While a good friend who is a hair stylist may know you well and have wonderful things to say about you, a letter from someone else who knows you well and has a more respected profession is probably going to look better. However, always remember to stick to people who know you well—that is more important than any status.

You will also need to be fingerprinted and/or have a criminal background check done. If your state requires fingerprints, you will be given a card or paperwork and be told to go to your local police station to be fingerprinted. A background check requires you to complete a form with your name, address, and Social Security number. This is then run through a computer to check for convictions, child abuse problems, or outstanding warrants.

If you have been arrested or convicted of a crime, all is not lost. The *Adoption and Safe Families Act* is a federal law that specifies which crimes states should screen for. Each state can opt out of these requirements and create their own, so it is important to check your state laws for specific information. In general, you are prohibited from adopting if you have been convicted (not just arrested) for any of the following.

Crimes against children, such as:
- child abuse or
- child neglect.

Felonies, consisting of:
- spousal abuse;
- crime against a child (such as child pornography);
- rape;
- sexual assault; or,
- homicide.

Felonies in the past five years, consisting of:
- physical assault or
- battery.

Drug-related offenses.

Keep in mind, there is generally a separate fee for the home study (which can range from $700 to $2000). If you are working with an agency, this may not be included in the agency fees.

Once you have jumped through all the required hoops, the social worker will write up a report that describes you and includes a recommendation as to whether or not you should adopt. The entire home study process can take anywhere from a few weeks to a few months, depending on how quickly things can be scheduled.

Ask to receive a copy of the complete home study. The home study will be valid for either a year or eighteen months. Most adoptions can be completed within that time frame.

Consent

All adoptions involve some form of *consent* — agreement by the birth parents that the child should be adopted. If there are no living birth parents or the child was abandoned, then consent must be given by the state or country where the child is a resident. Consent is the biggest and most important hurdle to adoption. Procedures are in place to make sure birth parents are given adequate time to make their decision.

The type of consent required varies in each state. The birth parents must sign a document in which they consent to the adoption and agree to give up all their rights to the child. In many states, the birth parents must also appear before a judge and verbally agree to the consent. Some states have the birth mother file a paper with the court called a *petition of relinquishment*. The birth mother can only give consent after the birth of the child, while the birth father can consent before birth. The thinking is that birth mothers often feel different after they have given birth to and have seen their child. (See the chart starting on page 125 for complete details on consent laws.)

The birth mother must always provide consent to the adoption. The birth father must also provide consent, if *paternity* has been established. Paternity can be established through an *admission* by the father or through a court proceeding. Many states also have what is called a *putative father registry*. This is a place where a man can register if he believes he is the father of a child. Before a child is placed for adoption, the putative father registry must be searched. If someone has registered, paternity will be tested.

Birth Fathers

Fathers' rights are an area of growing concern in the legal community. The problem with fathers' rights is that a birth father often does not know that he has fathered a child and the adoption happens without his knowledge or consent. The putative father registry helps with this issue, but does not completely alleviate it since if a man has no idea that a woman he was involved with became pregnant, he has no reason to register. Most men do not go and register every sexual encounter they have.

The *Baby Richard* case that occurred in Illinois is one many people think of when they think about the issue of fathers' rights. What many people do not understand about that case is that the birth mother lied to the birth father and told him the baby had died at birth, when instead she placed the baby for adoption. He later discovered the lie and eventually gained custody of the child who was, by that time, four years old. The birth mother also attempted to revoke her consent to the adoption. This case had components most cases do not — the marriage between the birth parents and the lie that was told.

Although the *Baby Richard* case is one that is unlikely to be repeated, it is a good example of why it is important to have consent from both birth parents whenever possible. In some instances that is not possible — and if your attorney is comfortable with the situation, then you should feel comfortable as well.

Older Children
In most states, older children that are adopted must give their consent. The age varies from state to state:

age 10:
- Alaska
- Arkansas
- Hawaii
- Maryland
- New Jersey
- New Mexico
- North Dakota

age 12:
- Arizona
- California
- Colorado
- Connecticut

- Florida
- Idaho
- Kentucky
- Massachusetts
- Montana
- New Hampshire
- North Carolina
- Ohio
- Oklahoma
- Pennsylvania
- South Dakota
- Texas
- Utah
- West Virginia

age 14:

- Alabama
- Delaware
- District of Columbia
- Georgia
- Illinois
- Indiana
- Iowa
- Kansas
- Maine
- Michigan
- Minnesota
- Mississippi
- Missouri
- Nebraska
- Nevada
- New York
- Oregon

- Rhode Island
- South Carolina
- Vermont
- Virginia
- Washington
- Wyoming

A child's consent is not required:
- Louisiana
- Tennessee
- Wisconsin

No Consent Needed

Consent is not needed if the birth parent has *abandoned* the child, had his or her rights *terminated* by the state (usually through an abuse or neglect proceeding in which the child is placed in foster care and then eventually freed up for adoption), is *dead*, or if there are *special circumstances*, such as failure of the parent to have contact with the child for a lengthy period of time. These situations normally occur when a child is in foster care and the state has terminated the parental rights. There are instances when a child can be placed for adoption by a birth mother and no consent will be needed from the birth father, if he has abandoned the child or had no contact with the child for a certain period of time, as specified in your state adoption laws.

When no consent is needed from the birth parents, the procedure seems as if it should go more quickly, but in reality it usually takes the same period of time. Adoptions are time consuming because of the amount of paperwork that must be processed about the adoptive parents and because many families are waiting to find a child to adopt. The consent process does not add that much time to the process. At the most it may add a month or two if there is an extended period after birth during which the birth mother can change her mind.

Notice

In some cases, the birth father may not be part of the child's life or may not be able to be located. In instances where this occurs, the court will allow *notice* to be given to him. This can include sending certified letters or court documents to his last known address or workplace or publishing a notice in a newspaper selected by the court. If the father does not respond, he is presumed to have waived his right to oppose the adoption. If notice is required in your adoption, your attorney will take careful steps to make sure it is done correctly. If notice is not given properly, the birth father could later come back and seek custody.

If notice is given properly and the birth father does not respond, his rights are terminated. Once parental rights are terminated, they can only be changed by showing that the proper procedure was not followed. If your state notice laws are carefully followed, there should not be problems with a birth father coming back later and trying to contest the adoption.

Timing of Consent

Birth fathers can give consent to adoption at any time. However, there are specific time frames in which a birth mother can give consent and have it be valid. This is usually only after the child is born. Alabama and Hawaii allow consent beforehand, but require a *reaffirmation* after the birth. There is usually a waiting period between the birth and when the birth mother's consent becomes final, and that can vary from twelve hours after the birth to fifteen days afterwards. (See Chapter 14 for more information about consent laws and timing.)

Consent Procedures

Birth parent consent can be done in writing (usually notarized) in some states. Other states require that it be done in court—either by appearing before the judge or by filing certain court papers. The birth parent must indicate that he or she understands the ramifications of what he or she is doing and willingly gives up all rights to the child.

The consent procedure is very simple when it occurs in court. The adoption case is scheduled for a court appearance. The birth mother appears and simply tells the court she consents to the adoption. The judge makes sure she understands exactly what she is agreeing to and that she is agreeing to it of her own volition. There is no trial or complicated hearing involved.

Revocation

Revocation is the withdrawal of consent by a birth parent. Everyone who is looking to adopt has heard horror stories about adoptions being revoked at the last minute. Revocation is actually difficult to do. A few states do not allow any revocation under any circumstances. Others permit revocation only if there has been fraud, coercion, or other factors that indicate that the birth parent did not have complete knowledge or free will at the time of the consent. A few states allow birth parents to change their minds for any reason within a certain time period.

If a birth mother revokes her consent, the adoption does not occur. Usually, if there is an agency involved, there will be last minute negotiations to try to complete the adoption, but by law, once a birth mother changes her mind, the adoptive family has no rights. The child is not theirs until the adoption is finalized and the adoption is not finalized without the completion of the consent.

While it is a sad thing to have happen, it is a possibility that all adoptive families must confront. The good news is that most birth mothers do not try to revoke their consent. To avoid a consent problem, it is important that the birth mother receive counseling during and after the pregnancy. It is also important that adoptive parents pursue only those adoptions that they have good feelings about and that seem likely to go through. If an adoption does fall through, you must know that it is not your fault and there is nothing you could have done to change the situation, as heartbreaking as it may be. You would not want to adopt a child knowing that you are taking him or her away from the birth mother against her will. Even if you believe that you can provide a better home for the child, you must accept the fact that the birth mother has the absolute right to keep her child if she so decides within the period of time allowed in your state. Once the court has finalized the adoption, there is no possibility that the adoption can be revoked. (Court proceedings are discussed later in this chapter.)

The following lists discuss when revocation is allowed and the time periods after consent for revocation in each state.

No revocation allowed (unless fraud, duress, etc.):
- Arizona
- California (agency adoption)
- Colorado
- Florida (if adoptive parents are identified)
- Kansas
- Mississippi
- Nebraska
- New Hampshire
- New Jersey
- New Mexico
- Oklahoma
- Oregon
- South Carolina
- Utah
- West Virginia
- Wisconsin
- Wyoming

No revocation at all (unless in the child's best interest):
- Hawaii
- Indiana
- Louisiana (birth fathers only)
- Massachusetts

- Nevada
- New York (private adoption)
- North Dakota
- Ohio
- Rhode Island

Three days:
- Florida (if adoptive parents not identified)
- Illinois
- Maine
- North Carolina (unborn infants and infants under three months of age)

Four days:
- Iowa

Five days (after birth):
- Louisiana

Seven days:
- North Carolina

Ten days:
- Alaska
- Arkansas
- District of Columbia
- Georgia
- Minnesota
- Tennessee

Fourteen days:
- Alabama

Fifteen days:
- Oklahoma (out-of-court consents only)
- Virginia

Twenty days:
- Kentucky

Twenty-one days:
- Vermont

Thirty days:
- California (direct placement)
- Maryland

Forty-five days:
- New York (consent made outside of court)

Sixty days:
- Delaware

Any time before final decree:
- Connecticut
- Idaho
- Michigan
- Missouri
- Montana
- Pennsylvania
- South Dakota (final decree takes two years)
- Washington

Adoptive Parent Consent

It is also important to understand that the adoptive parents must give their consent to the adoption. You can change your mind any time until the adoption is finalized by the court. This is something very few adoptive families consider, but it is important to understand your rights. Just because you say you want to adopt a child, you are not obligated to do so. However, if you change your mind, you cannot get a refund on the expenses you have paid. If you adopt a child and later determine that the situation is not going to work, you cannot just give the child back. You need to have your parental rights terminated by the state and you will also probably be required to pay for the expenses of foster care up until termination.

Adoption Court Procedures

The actual court procedure for an adoption is the last big hurdle in the process. As previously discussed, revocation of consent is the only real worry facing prospective adoptive parents at this point.

Your adoption will be handled in your state's family, juvenile, or surrogate's court. Your attorney will file your adoption petition and other paperwork. The court will review all the documents, including the home study and background checks. If the birth parents are required to or choose to give consent in front of the judge, this will happen in the courtroom. If the child is of the age set by the state, he or she will be asked to consent to the adoption. If a birth father could not be located and notice was given, the court will review the notice to make sure it meets the state's requirements. The adoptive parents appear in court to tell the court they agree to the adoption. The adoption is then finalized and the judge signs the final order. This makes it official and legal.

There is no testimony, cross-examination, or other courtroom theatrics. Adoption procedures are quiet and simple. There are legalities that must be taken care of, but by the time you go to court to finalize the adoption, all problems should be behind you. Once you have dealt with the consent issues, your adoption is usually very simple.

Adoption proceedings are happy occasions and judges are usually pleased to be part of them. Judges spend most of their time dealing with cases where people are arguing or are unhappy, so it is a pleasant experience for them to handle a case where the result is a happy ending. Most judges will allow family and friends to join you in the courtroom. The court staff will often congratulate the adoptive parents and "ooh" and "ahh" over the adoptive child. When the adoptive child is old enough to speak and understand what is happening, he or she is often made a part of the proceeding as well and is made to feel as if something very special has happened for him or her. Some judges will even give the child a certificate or a card in further recognition of how special the event is. If you wish to take photographs, be sure to check with the court staff beforehand.

Postplacement

With most agency adoptions, you will have some *postplacement* contact with the agency or with a social worker. You may have one or two postplacement visits from the social worker to make sure things are going smoothly and to offer some assistance with adjustments. These visits are usually nothing to worry about. The worker is not going to rip your child from your arms and take him or her back. The worker will prepare a postplacement report that is filed with the agency and may be filed with the court if required in your state.

NOTE: *A child may be placed with you before the adoption is finalized. This happens because a birth mother gives birth and knows she wants to place the child, but it takes time for the actual finalization to occur.*

Postplacement visits are not about determining if the adoption should be allowed. They are about making sure you have support and helping the agency see that it went well. Postplacement visits cannot undo an adoption; however, if a worker notices a child is being neglected or abused, it could open up a court procedure to deal with the situation. Once your state has finalized and legalized your adoption, you have nothing to worry about unless a postplacement visit is required before finalization in your state.

Birth Certificates

After the adoption is finalized, you need to get an amended birth certificate for your adopted child. Your attorney will request this form. The new birth certificate will list the adoptive parents, but maintain the child's birth date. This will be your child's official, legal birth certificate. The old birth certificate still exists as a state record, but it is not accessible. The adoption court proceeding also becomes sealed and not accessible.

> **From the Expert**
>
> Many states now have their adoption forms online. Check your state court system's website for your state's forms. For example, you can see New York's forms at:
>
> **www.courts.state.ny.us/ forms/familycourt/ adoption.shtml**

This is why you hear about adult adoptees having difficulty finding their birth parents. The information about the birth becomes inaccessible to protect privacy.

If you are interested in an adoption where information about the birth parents is accessible to the child, information is available later in this book. (See Chapter 2 for more information about open adoptions.)

Adoption Financial Credits

Once you adopt, under the *Hope for Children Act*, you are entitled to up to a $10,000 deduction (as of the time this book was published) for the expenses associated with your adoption that you have not been reimbursed for on your income tax return. If you adopt a special needs child, you are entitled to the full deduction (with some income restrictions) without having to show expenses. Additionally, if you cannot take the full deduction, you can *carry forward* (take in later years) the remaining amounts. Talk to your accountant or tax preparer about this credit. (Second-parent adoptions do not qualify.)

Additionally, once your child has been adopted, you can list him or her as a dependant on your federal taxes, so make sure you let your tax preparer know about the adoption. Some states also offer adoption tax cred-

---

From the Expert

If your company does not currently offer an adoption assistance program, information about starting one is available through:

The Adoption-Friendly Workplace Program
877-777-4222
www.adoptionfriendly workplace.org

---

its, so inquire about this. Once you are a parent, there are other child-related tax breaks available, including deductions for child care. Sit down with your tax preparer and find out how you can best approach taxes as a new parent.

Many employers offer adoption expense reimbursement (a survey found that 98% of the top 837 US employers provided some kind of assistance). Check with your human resource manager to find out if your company offers such a program. Employer assistance is not taxed, so this is yet another tax break.

Family Leave

The federal *Family and Medical Leave Act* allows parents to take unpaid time off from work to care for a newly adopted child (as well as ill family members and for the birth of biological children) within the first twelve months after placement of the child.

NOTE: *The Act will only apply to children that are your own, so taking time off before your adoption is finalized is not covered under the Act, unless you have some other reason you can use for taking the time (caring for yourself or another family member).*

You must work for an employer with at least fifty employees and you must have been employed at least twelve months and worked at least 1250 hours. You can take up to twelve total weeks leave in a twelve-month period. If you and your spouse work for the same employer, you are only given twelve weeks total between you to split. You can take all the leave at once or spread the leave out so that you work some or all of the time on a part time basis. When possible, you must give thirty days notice of the leave. When you return to work, your employer must reinstate you to your job or to a similar position.

Some states also have family leave laws, so be sure to check with your human resource manager to determine if you are entitled to additional state leave. The states that currently have state family leave acts are:

- California
- Connecticut
- District of Columbia
- Hawaii
- Maine
- Minnesota
- New Jersey
- Oregon
- Rhode Island
- Vermont
- Washington
- Wisconsin

Additionally, California has a state disability law that says that parents of newborns, as well as parents of newly adopted children of any age, qualify for a disability leave that provides the new parents with a percentage of their pay as well as job security. You may also qualify for paid maternity or paternity leave or special adoption leave under your company's policies.

Insurance and Planning for the Future

Once the child is placed with you, you can contact your health insurance company about adding the child to your policy. You will need to have family coverage to add your child. If you do not have family coverage, you may need to wait until the next enrollment period (which usually occurs four times per year) to change your coverage to family coverage. If you have family coverage already, contact your insurer before the adoption is finalized and ask what you need to do to have the child added. You want to be sure your child is covered from the moment of the adoption forward, so this means starting the paperwork before the adoption is completed.

Life Insurance

If you do not already have life insurance, it is a good idea to consider purchasing some. If you are married, you will probably want to name your spouse as beneficiary. If you are unmarried, you will want to name your child as beneficiary. Some parents also like to purchase life insurance for their new child, but it is often a better idea to create an investment account for the child.

You may also wish to consider creating a 529 College Savings Account for your child to help defray the expenses of a college education. There are many options and it is important to create a complete financial plan for your family. Talk to your financial planner.

Wills

You will also want to have a will drawn up. Once you adopt a child, he or she inherits from you through the laws of your state, so a will is not important for that reason. It is important because in your will you can name a guardian who would have custody of your child should you die (and if your spouse or partner should also die). When choosing a guardian, be sure to choose someone who has similar beliefs as yours and who will be close to your child. Be sure to talk this decision over with the potential guardian. If the guardian you name is unable or unwilling to take on the responsibility of guardianship, the court will find a replacement among your family members, but you want to have a hand in this decision. Name an alternate guardian in case something happens to your first choice.

From the Expert
Read your state's adoption laws at:
www.law.cornell.edu/ topics/Table_Adoption.htm

Chapter 17

Second-Parent Adoption

Second-parent adoptions are often referred to as *stepparent adoptions*. The child lives with one legal parent and the child's other parent may be deceased, completely out of touch, or without custody. This legal parent remarries and the stepparent wishes to adopt the child. These adoptions are quite common and are generally simpler than other kinds of adoptions.

If a stepparent does not adopt the child, he or she might have an important parental role in the child's life, but in the eyes of the law, he or she has no authority over or legal connection to the child. The child cannot inherit from the stepparent (unless the stepparent leaves something to him or her in a will) or receive any survivor benefits from the stepparent. The stepparent cannot make medical decisions or educational decisions for the child (unless specifically authorized by the parent) and if the stepparent and the legal parent divorce or break up, the stepparent has no legal right to spend time with the child or seek custody or visitation. Additionally, if the legal parent dies, the stepparent would not automatically be named as the child's guardian or be given custody.

Stepparents often assume a parental role in the child's life, but are lacking any kind of legal role. A stepparent or second-parent adoption legalizes the role the stepparent already has in the child's life.

Deciding to Adopt a Stepchild
The decision to adopt a stepchild should not be made lightly. Once you adopt your stepchild, he or she is your child and the adoption cannot be

undone (although in some states there is a short window in which con-sent to the adoption can be withdrawn). You will be financially and legally responsible for the child and should you get divorced, you could be liable for child support. A stepchild who is adopted becomes your legal child in all ways.

A stepchild that you adopt is able to inherit from you. If you have other children, this adopted stepchild will be treated exactly the same as your other children when it comes to inheritance. Sometimes this can cause bad feelings in families. If you want your adopted stepchild to be treated differently, it is important that you have a will made specifying what you want to leave to each child.

If the child's other parent is deceased, the adoption might be an emo-tional issue for the child. Some children are resistant to the idea of a step-parent replacing the deceased parent and want to reserve a special role for that parent. In this kind of situation, it is a good idea to explore the child's feelings and possibly seek some family counseling to help sort it out. It may take some time for the child to be ready to take this step. Some stepparents never adopt their stepchildren and there is nothing wrong with that choice either.

Another stumbling block in second-parent adoptions is the way the legal parent and the stepparent feel. Some stepparents are hesitant to take on a legal role in the child's life. Particularly if they do not have biologi-cal children of their own, some stepparents feel unsure about the respon-sibilities of parenthood. It can also be daunting to feel as if you are taking over for a parent who is deceased or out of the picture.

In other situations, the marriage might be experiencing some trouble and the parent and stepparent might see the adoption as providing some additional glue to help hold it together. It is important to understand that a stepparent adoption is not a quick fix for marital problems.

A newly married couple might feel as if they need to hurry to do a stepparent adoption in order to make their new family complete. However, it may simply be too soon in the relationship for the adoption to feel right for the child and everyone else involved.

If you have other children and you are adopting your stepchild, you need to consider the feelings of your children. Some children feel that the adopted child will somehow usurp their positions. It is similar to the way a child feels when a sibling is born into the family, but is more intense because your children clearly know that this new child is not related to you or the rest of the family in quite the same way. Taking some time to help your existing children accept the adoption will help everyone adjust. It is a good idea to have open and frank discussions with everyone in the family about the adoption. Family counseling can help you work through many problems.

If you adopt a stepchild, your parents become your adopted child's grandparents. This can go smoothly or cause some problems. If you have been married to the child's parent for a long time, the child has probably already established a relationship with your parents. If this is a relatively new situation, it may take some time. Regardless of how things have been up to this point, it is important that your parents understand that this child is now fully and completely yours, and by extension, theirs. They should work hard to make sure they treat all of their grandchildren equally or there is sure to be resentment.

It is important that second-parent adoptions are done for the right reason—to solidify a relationship that has already been established between the stepparent and the child and to provide legal rights to the child and stepparent.

Qualifications to Adopt

If you are married to the child's legal parent, you can seek a second-parent adoption. In some states you do not have to be married, but can simply be partners. (See Chapter 22 for information about same-sex couples.) It is usually best to wait until you have been married at least one year before seeking to adopt your stepchild. This demonstrates to the court that you have had time to establish a close relationship with the child and that your marriage is stable (some states require this).

Notice or Consent

The parent that has custody of the child must consent to the adoption and in some states must actually readopt the child as well (so that you are adopting the child together as a couple). While this seems silly, it is simply a formality and does nothing to change the relationship between the child and the existing parent.

If your stepchild has another legal or biological parent that is alive, then that parent is entitled to some kind of notice of the adoption and the chance to deny consent. This other parent must consent to give up all rights to the child or fail to respond to the legal notice that is given in order for the adoption to occur. This legal notice is done by giving the parent papers explaining the intention to adopt the child. In some states these documents can be mailed to the parent or personally *served* (given to him or her in person by a process server). If the other parent cannot be located, you may need to go through a process in which the notice is published in a newspaper.

Stepparent adoption is also possible when the parent has had his or her parental rights terminated by the court (such as in an abuse or neglect situation). In some states, if the other parent does not give consent, his or her rights can be terminated in certain circumstances, for example, if he or she has not had any contact with the child for a long period of time.

If you give the biological parent notice and he or she does not consent, the only way to get around it is to prove neglect and have his or her parental rights terminated or to show the parent has abandoned the child. There is no way to force a biological parent to agree to an adoption, even if the adoption would clearly be in the best interest of the child. If you are in a situation where the biological parent will not consent and you cannot find a way to terminate rights, remember that being a parent is really a state of mind. You can think of yourself as the child's parent and act like his or her parent even if the law will not recognize you as such. Some families that have confronted this problem act as if the stepparent is really a parent. Once the child is an adult, you can legally adopt him or her then to make it official. What makes a parent is what one does, not what a piece of paper says.

Preadoption Procedures

Some states waive the requirement of a home study in second-parent adoptions; some states have laws that require it, but permit judges to waive it; and, other states require stepparents (and the child's existing parent if he or she must also adopt the child) to go through the home study and background check process. Usually when a home study is required, the primary focus will be on the stepparent, his or her history, how long they have been married, and what kind of relationship he or she has with the child. However, when it is required, the home study process is usually minimal. The state department of social services usually performs the home study when it is required.

The states that do not require home studies for second-parent adoptions include:

- Alabama
- Alaska
- Arizona
- California
- Colorado
- Connecticut
- Florida
- Georgia
- Maryland
- Michigan
- Minnesota
- Mississippi
- Nebraska
- Ohio
- Pennsylvania
- South Carolina
- Texas

The areas where home studies can be waived for second-parent adoptions include:

- Arizona
- District of Columbia
- Missouri
- Nevada
- New Hampshire
- Oklahoma
- Oregon
- Utah

Second-Parent Adoption Process

Stepparent adoptions can be handled on your own without an attorney more easily than other types of adoption, although it is a good idea to hire an attorney to ensure that the case is handled properly. Some states require representation by an attorney.

If you do choose to handle the adoption on your own, you need to contact the court in your state that does adoptions to obtain forms and get information about the filing procedures.

A second-parent adoption follows the same procedure as any other adoption, with the only difference being the home study is sometimes not required. (See Chapter 16 for more details on adoption procedures.)

In many states when a second parent adopts the child, the biological parent that he or she is married to must also adopt the child, so that both people must complete the paperwork. This does nothing to change the biological parent's status and is simply an antiquated procedure. It used to be that only married couples could adopt a child. Some states still require that the second-parent adoption be done by both parents so that both names go through the entire process and both names end up on the birth certificate at the end of the process.

Chapter 18

Domestic Agency Adoption

Most people who adopt use an agency to help them locate a birth mother or a child, and to help process the adoption. If you are adopting a child born in the United States, the agency you use will be a *domestic agency*. Domestic agencies are not all alike. The first important distinction is between public and private agencies. A *public agency* refers to a state department of social services or department of family and children's services. These agencies handle the adoption of children who were in foster care and have been freed for adoption by the state's courts or who have been surrendered by their birth parents. Most of these children are not babies and many are special needs children. There are many children available for adoption through these state agencies.

Private agencies are those run by private entities. Some are nonprofit, while others are for-profit businesses. Some are run by religious organizations, while others are nonsectarian. You will find that there is a wide selection of private agencies to choose from.

Public Agencies

Public agency adoptions have the same requirements as other types of adoptions, including the home study, background check, and court procedure to finalize the adoption. Public agency adoptions are usually the fastest and least expensive type of adoption. However, since the children tend to be older, the transition and adjustment period is often more difficult.

All children that are available for adoption in a state are shown in the state's photolisting book. The books show a photo and description of each child.

There are several ways to adopt a child through a public agency.

Foster Care

The *foster care* system is set up to provide a home for children who have been removed from their homes because of abuse, neglect, and occasionally due to juvenile delinquency. Children who have been abandoned or voluntarily placed with the state by parents are also placed in foster care. These children are placed in the temporary care of the state while their parents deal with the court system or the court determines that their parents abandoned them. Many times these children are returned to their parents if the court decides that no abuse or neglect occurred or if the parents meet the requirements set up by the agency (such as counseling, child care classes, maintaining a stable lifestyle, and so on) and the parents are deemed fit to care for the children.

> **From the Expert**
> Find contacts for foster care agencies in your state at:
> **www.fosterparenting.com**
>
> and click on the "Foster" tab.
>
> Get support and information about foster care adoption at:
> **www.DaveThomas FoundationforAdoption.org**

In other instances, the children never return home. Most states now make an effort to move the case through the court system quickly so that the children are either returned home or are freed for adoption and do not languish in foster care for years. The federal *Adoption and Safe Families Act* states that if a child has been in foster care for at least fifteen months or if his or her parents abandoned the child, the parental rights can be terminated and the child can be freed for adoption. For the children that do not return home, the court severs the biological parents' ties to the children and frees them for adoption.

Many adoptions occur by the foster parents who care for the children while their case is pending or while their parents are trying to meet the agency's requirements for return. Becoming a foster parent is one route to public agency adoption. To become a foster parent, you must first identify the private agencies that contract for foster care with the state. In most states, the public agency itself does not directly handle foster care placement. Prospective foster care parents must work with a public agency that handles the state agency's contract for foster care.

To become a foster parent you must:
• complete a series of classes;
• provide financial, personal, and health information about yourself and your family;
• be able to provide appropriate housing for a child or children;
• be prepared for ongoing contact with caseworkers; and,
• understand that a foster care parent's job is to care for the child, while helping to reunite him or her with the biological parents. (Adoption is not an option until the child has been freed for adoption.)

When you become a foster parent, you will make yourself available to children who may or may not be freed for adoption. At the time of initial placement, you have no way of knowing how the case will ultimately be resolved. As a foster parent, you will receive a small monthly stipend that is meant to cover the child's expenses and you will also have to follow the caseworker's instructions. While you are the foster care parent, the child is in the custody of the state and the caseworker will have absolute authority over major decisions involving the child. Foster parents have very little rights when it comes to the children they care for.

Contact your local public agency for information about which private agencies handle foster care and how you can apply.

Legal Risk Placement

Legal risk placement occurs when you accept a child that you would like to adopt who has not yet been completely freed for adoption. The intent of the placement is for the child to begin to develop a relationship with you and to begin to put down roots. However, the child is not legally free for adoption yet and something may happen that could prevent the adoption from happening. While you are waiting for the child to be freed for adoption, you are acting as a foster care parent since the state has custody and control of the child. This kind of placement allows you to get a jump on the whole process by bonding with your child before the finalization, but you must accept the risk that the adoption may not be finalized.

Traditional Adoption

Another method of adopting a child through a public agency is the traditional method, where the child is not placed until the adoption is complete. The child remains in foster care until the legal process is finalized and then comes home to the adoptive parents. This is the least risky of all the public agency adoption choices, but it can also be the most emotionally difficult for a child old enough to understand what is happening. There is no transition period as there is in foster care placement or legal risk placement.

Public Agency Adoption Issues

When adopting a child through a public agency, make sure to obtain full medical records and family histories if available. Before you agree to the adoption, you want to get as much information as you can. The child may have a history or background that does not work for you. (It is important to be honest and face the fact that not every child is the right child for you.) The caseworkers who manage the child while he or she is in foster care have access to the biological parents and can obtain this information. They can also provide infor-

> ### From the Expert
> Find your state public adoption agency online at:
> **http://naic.acf.hhs.gov/ general/nad/index.cfm**

mation about assessments and evaluations that have been done while the child
has been in foster care.

Because the child is usually leaving
parents that are alive and have some
kind of relationship with the child (no
matter how dysfunctional), there are
significant transition issues for the child

> **From the Expert**
>
> Get tips on helping an older child deal with adoption at:
>
> **www.familyhelper.net/ arc/old.html**

and the adoptive parent. If the child is old enough, he or she will remember his or her biological parents and will have some kind of attachment
to them, even if they were terrible parents. It takes a lot of time and
patience to help children adjust. It also takes time for them to learn to
trust adoptive parents. Many of these children were abused, malnour-
ished, or emotionally damaged.

Moving into a loving, nurturing home can be a shock. Some adoptive
parents report that their new children would raid the refrigerator and
gorge—certain that soon they would starve again. Other children have
been known to steal from new family members or harm new siblings.
There are numerous behavioral issues you might face after the adoption.
A good counselor or therapist is essential to help everyone make a
smooth adjustment. Your social worker from the agency can provide
some help with adjustment or can recommend a private counselor. It is
also a good idea to get involved with an adoption support group.

Special Needs

Many public agency adoptive children have special needs. Special needs
children are those that take longer to place and include:

- school-age children or teens;
- children with physical, mental, or emotional disabilities;
- sibling groups that must stay together; and,
- children of certain racial or ethnic groups that are difficult to place.

Simply because a child is described as special needs does not mean that
there is anything wrong with him or her. It just means that this child is one

that is difficult to place. Your home might be the perfect place for a special needs child. For this reason it is important to find out what evaluations have been done, what the specialists recommend, and what kind of care or treatment the child needs.

Learn about the child's exposure to or use of drugs or alcohol and have a treatment plan in place to deal with these issues. Get detailed information about the child's behavior and where he or she has lived and who has cared for him or her in the past. Ask for copies of all reports, evaluations, and assessments.

Special needs children may appeal to people who do not wish to care for a baby or toddler, or who have special skills dealing with disabled children or in working with teens. Additionally, special needs children are sometimes easier to adopt because the agency is willing to overlook certain problems with the adoptive family in order to help the children find a home.

Adopting a special needs child can be a challenge, but it can also be tremendously rewarding. Special needs kids often recognize the fact that they are hard to place. Sometimes the adjustment process can be difficult because they tend to erect barriers since they have had their hopes dashed so many times in the past. Adopting a special needs child does not work for everyone, but many families find it to be rewarding.

From the Expert

The *National Resource Center for Special Needs Adoption* can provide information and support for those adopting special needs children. Contact them at:

National Resource Center for Special Needs Adoption
16250 Northland Drive
Suite 120
Southfield, MI 48075
248-443-0306
**www.nrcadoption.org/
index.htm**

Other sites that can provide information include:
**www.special-needs.
adoption.com**
and
www.spaulding.org

Financial Assistance for Public Agency Adoptions

Because of the difficult nature of many public agency adoptions and because many of the children adopted do have special needs, there is special funding available to assist the parents in caring for the child after the adoption.

Title IV-E Assistance

Special needs children may qualify for federal funding assistance. The child may be receiving Social Security Insurance (SSI) payments already, but may also qualify for *Adoption and Safe Families Act* (ASFA) funding. ASFA provides financial assistance for children who are adopted and:

> **From the Expert**
> For more information about state subsidies, visit:
> **www.adopting.org/ subsidy.html**

- were receiving Temporary Assistance to Needy Families (TANF) in other words, welfare, in the birth home or
- were eligible for SSI in the birth home which means they were disabled and were in a home that met certain financial requirements.

When you are negotiating your adoption with your public agency, you need to ask about eligibility for this funding. You can apply directly through your local social services or family services department. Usually the social worker who handles your adoption will help you apply.

Adoption Assistance Agreement

An *adoption assistance agreement* is a contract between the adoptive parents and the state agency, describing the ongoing monthly payments the state will make to the parents after the adoption is complete to help with the expense of raising the child. The payments are often for a few hundred dollars per month.

The agreement is made before the adoption takes place and is in effect as long as the child is a minor. The agreement may also include provisions

> **From the Expert**
>
> For information on what your state pays for adoption assistance, see:
>
> **www.nacac.org/subsidy_ stateprofiles.html**

for assistance with the child's medical expenses (see the Medicaid section later in this chapter). Some states include additional funding amounts for children that are especially difficult to care for. These are known as Level of Care (LOC) payments.

These agreements are common for special needs adoptions where the child is known to need continuing care or services that are outside of the normal medical needs children experience. They are provided so that families will adopt these children and not have to worry about affording the care the child will need.

The agreement is enforceable. If there is future disagreement about it, an administrative hearing is held to resolve the problem. Do not finalize your adoption until this document is signed.

If you negotiate an agreement, make sure it:

- is in writing;
- contains beginning and ending dates for the payments;
- specifies the amount of payments and any changes to the amount as the child ages;
- does not put excessive restrictions or requirements on you after the adoption occurs;
- specifies the reporting or certification you need to comply with to continue to receive payments;
- lists all services to be provided by the state;
- explains how subsidies or services can be increased or decreased and what kind of notice is required;
- describes Medicaid coverage for the child;
- explains what happens if you move out of state or if both adoptive parents die;
- describes what you need to do to get an administrative hearing should you need one; and,
- takes into account your child's needs and your family's situation.

Medicaid

A special needs child may qualify for Medicaid. The state Medicaid program will pay many of his or her medical expenses both before and after the adoption. If you have a family health care policy, your child can also receive

> **From the Expert**
>
> For more information about Medicaid, visit:
>
> **www.cms.hhs.gov/ medicaid**

treatment under that plan—it may cover some of the things that Medicaid does not. Medicaid is a federal program, but is administered by each state individually with different rights and procedures in each state. Your social worker will provide information about your child's Medicaid eligibility.

Tax Credits

Parents adopting a special needs child are entitled to a $10,000 tax credit, without having to show any expenses. This applies to families earning under $150,000 per year. Those earning between $150,000 and $189,999 receive a reduced credit in proportion to income. This is a credit that is nonrefundable—meaning that you cannot get money refunded above your tax liability. But if you do have a lower income, you can claim the credit over a five-year period so that you can use more of it. There are also some state tax credits available, also you should check with your tax preparer to find out what your state provides. (See Chapter 16 for more information about tax credits.)

For the purposes of the tax credit, a special needs child is one who cannot be placed with adoptive parents without providing a subsidy. A reasonable, but unsuccessful effort must be made to place the child for adoption without a subsidy, unless it is in the child's best interests to remain with prospective adoptive parents with whom they have significant emotional ties. Factors or conditions related to the

> **From the Expert**
>
> IRS Publication 968 explains tax credits in more details. Find it at:
>
> **www.irs.gov**

From the Expert

For information and resources about special education, visit:

www.seriweb.com

The federal *Department of Education* has a section about special education located at:
www.ed.gov/about/offices/ list/osers/osep/index.html

Wrights Law is an excellent site devoted to helping parents navigate the system. Find it at:
www.wrightslaw.com

The *National Dissemination Center for Children with Disabilities* is another excellent resource. Find it at:
www.nichcy.org

From the Expert

Some states provide special tuition assistance or waivers for foster care children who have been adopted. For information, see:

www.nacac.org/subsidy factsheets/tuition.html

---

special needs determination may include ethnic background, age, membership in a minority or sibling group, the presence of a medical condition, or physical, mental, or emotional disabilities.

Other Assistance

Organizations for parents of special needs children (including those referenced earlier in this chapter) will provide support and assistance as you adopt and raise a special needs child. If your child is of school-age, or will soon be of school-age, you will need to begin to learn your way around the special education process.

Biological Relatives

Another important issue is the child's *biological relatives*. While a court can sever legal ties between a child and his or her biological family, the court cannot change the emotional ties that exist when an older child is adopted. For this reason, some courts permit adoptive parents and biological relatives of the child to create and record kinship agreements. These agreements set out a plan for how the child will continue to have contact with important family members (such as grandparents, siblings, aunts and uncles). This prevents a child from feeling totally cutoff from his or her family and ethnic heritage. (See Chapter 14 for more information about kinship agreements.)

Agency Liability

All agencies have a duty to fully disclose information about the child being placed for adoption. This duty is particularly important when working with a public agency, since most children placed through it have had difficult home lives or suffer disabilities. The agency must disclose to you:

- how and why the child came into the state's care;
- why the child remained in the care of the state;
- why the parental rights were terminated; and,
- why the agency decided to place the child.

It is also important that the case worker explain to you the causal relationship that exists between a child's home life and his or her behavior — how the things he or she went through have caused him or her to act the way he or she does and how it might impact future behavior. The caseworker is responsible for reading the entire file and disclosing all the information in it to you. Failure to do so is negligence on the part of the agency.

There is some dispute about how far a worker must go. Some states say that a caseworker should make reasonable efforts to investigate the background of the family the child came from, while most states say that the agency is not required to take investigative steps.

The child's file should include the following:

- hospital records;
- records from doctor's offices;
- the child's HIV history (including testing);
- school records; and,
- what family background is known.

An agency that fails to disclose all of this information can be sued for *wrongful adoption*. Some agencies in the past have placed a child and lied about his or her history or purposefully failed to disclose important information. When a court finds that wrongful adoption has occurred, money damages are awarded. These damages can be *punitive* (to punish the agency) and can also be *compensatory*, to pay back the family for the medical or psychological care it has had to pay that it did not anticipate. Sometimes damages are also awarded to pay the family back for physical harm caused by the adoptive child (if, for example, the child has caused damage to property or harmed family members). The family cannot recover the ordinary costs of raising a child. In a few rare cases, the family has been allowed to dissolve the adoption and return the child to the agency.

The best way to avoid these kinds of problems is to insist on complete disclosure, to go over documents carefully, and to use an adoption attorney who will help you make sure your rights are protected.

Private Agency Adoption

Private agencies have infants as well as older children to place for adoption. An infant will take the longest to adopt (because you may need to wait for one to be born), while older children are placed more quickly. Most parents using private agencies are looking for babies.

Evaluating A Private Agency

The first step to working with a private agency is to carefully select one. Since you will pay an application fee, it is usually not a good idea to apply to more than one agency at a time. Be sure to evaluate agencies carefully. (See Chapter 15 for more information about this.)

Once you have narrowed down your search to a few agencies, talk to the adoption specialist at your state department of social services. He or she can tell you what the agencies are like and what kind of information the state has available about them. Check with the Better Business Bureau in your state to determine if any complaints have been filed against the agency. Talk with other adoptive parents and find out what they have heard about the agency.

Fees

Compare the home study costs and other fees that each agency charges. Less might not always be better if you feel a more expensive agency does a better job. Be absolutely certain that the

> ### From the Expert
> To find a list of private agencies in your area to search for licensed adoption agencies in your state, visit the *National Adoption Information Clearinghouse* website at:
> **www.adoptuskids.org**

agency and the social worker who does the home study are licensed in your state. Most states do not set limits on the fees an agency may charge, but do require that they must not exceed what is considered *reasonable and customary*. Cost can range anywhere from $4000 to $30,000, depending on the agency. Agencies run by religious groups tend to cost less. Some agencies charge a flat fee, while others charge for each service separately. Be sure to get a complete list of what is covered by a flat fee.

The following are fees typically charged and the average cost of each. Your costs may be higher or lower but this list gives a rough estimate of what to expect to pay in fees. The average costs include:

- application—$250;
- home study—$1200;
- post placement services—$500;
- psychological evaluations of parents—$200 each;
- physical exams for parents—$75 each;
- document fees—varies (often $1000);
- court fees and legal costs—varies by state (up to $12,000);
- advertising fees—$2000;
- birth mother living costs—varies;
- medical expenses for mother and baby—varies;
- legal fees for birth mother may be $1000; and,
- counseling—$1000.

Be sure to compare fees between several agencies so that you have an understanding of what the average fees are like in your area.

You may be asked to pay for most expenses up front or you may be able to pay for them as they occur. Find out how the agency requires you to pay before applying.

Expenses

Be skeptical if the agency takes money paid for your birth mother's expenses and places it in an escrow pool out of which it pays all birth mothers' individual expenses for placing babies with the agency. With this method, you do not pay your birth mother's actual expenses, but instead pay an average cost that takes into account high expenses some birth mothers have. Most states require an accounting be made to the court, listing the expenses the adoptive parents have paid for.

Because most of the babies available for placement have not been born yet, there is the very real chance that the birth mother will change her mind before placement occurs. Always find out what the agency's policy is about the fees you have already paid — can you roll them over to use for another birth mother should the birth mother you choose change her mind? Idaho is the only state that requires birth parents to reimburse adoptive parents if the birth parents change their minds and decide not to place the child for adoption.

Some states permit adoptive parents to pay for the birth mother's living expenses during her pregnancy. Adoptive parents pay for the medical expenses of both birth mother and baby. The baby will not be covered by your health insurance plan until the child is placed with you, so these expenses are out-of-pocket expenses for adoptive parents, unless the birth mother has health insurance coverage (or the adoptive parents purchase a policy for her).

Many adoptive parents feel a need to give the birth mother a gift after the birth. While this may seem like a wonderful gesture, it in fact can cause problems for you since many states prohibit any compensation to the birth mother for the adoption. This is intended to prevent the buying and selling of babies, but also prevents extravagant gifts. Small tokens of appreciation may be acceptable, but you need to check with your agency and your attorney before doing anything. (See Chapter 20 for more information about the length of time living expenses can be paid.)

The following states specifically list certain expenses adoptive parents cannot pay or cap the payments:

- Connecticut ($1500 limit);
- Delaware (nothing other than court and legal expenses);
- Idaho ($2000 limit);
- Illinois (does not allow lost wages, gifts, and educational expenses);
- Indiana ($3000 limit);
- Iowa (nothing other than room and board and counseling);
- Kentucky (does not allow for payment of birth parents' attorney fees);
- Maine (nothing other than legal costs, counseling, transportation to services, foster care, and living expenses);
- Minnesota (does not allow for lost wages, gifts, or educational expenses);
- Montana (does not allow for education, vehicle, salary, wages, vacations, or permanent housing for birth mother);
- New Hampshire (no gifts over $50 or educational expenses);
- New Mexico (nothing other than living expenses, medical costs, travel expenses, counseling, and legal/court fees);
- Ohio (nothing other than medical costs and legal expenses);
- Utah (nothing other than legal fees and expenses, medical care, maternity expenses, and living expenses); and,
- Wisconsin (does not permit lost wages or living expenses or anything other than counseling, maternity clothes, medical care, legal fees, birthing classes, and a $50 gift).

Interstate Issues

Depending on what state you live in, you may find that there are not many children available to adopt from within your state. If this is the case, you may need to adopt a child that is born in another state. To do so, you and the agency must be in compliance with the *Interstate*

Compact, a federal law that governs how children are transported between states for adoption purposes. Each state has an Interstate Compact administrator. The administrators in the state you live in and the state you are adopting from must both agree to the adoption. Your adoption agency and attorney will handle this technicality for you.

Ethnic Concerns

You also need to be aware of a federal law called the *Multiethnic Placement Act.* It denies federal funding to adoption agencies that delay or deny placement because of race (in other words, wait to place a child only with parents of the same race as the child). If you are interested in adopting a child with an ethnic background that is different than yours, ask if the agency complies with this statute. If you believe you have been denied a placement due to race, talk to your adoption attorney or contact your state attorney general.

> **From the Expert**
>
> For support in raising a multiethnic family, contact the *Association of Multiethnic Americans* at:
>
> **www.ameasite.org/ ipride_.html**

Chapter 19

International Adoption

International adoption is the adoption of a child from a country outside the US. International adoption has become more popular in recent years with publicity about how many waiting children there are in countries around the world. International adoption is an excellent choice if you do not want to wait to find a birth mother or new baby and do not mind adopting a child who is not a newborn. The procedure is not as complicated as some people expect it to be and the costs end up being about the same when you factor in travel expenses. The procedure is similar to those for domestic adoptions but involves extra steps such as dealing with the United States Department of Homeland Security's Citizenship and Immigration Services (USCIS)—once known as the Immigration and Naturalization Service (INS)—and US and overseas courts.

From the Expert

The *Joint Council of International Children's Services* has a list of agencies it accredits that can be found at:
www.jcics.org

The *International Adoption Consortium* also has a similar list that can be found at:
www.welcomegarden.com/ resources_by_state.html

For more information on choosing an international adoption agency, see:
www.adopting.org/ choosagn.html

From the Expert

You can search for agencies by the country you wish to adopt from or by the state you live in at:

http://directory. adoption.com

Choosing an Agency

You will always need to work with an agency to do an international adoption, since children are available only through agencies in foreign countries. Some private agencies handle only domestic adoption or only international adoption, while others handle both types. To find an agency, check with your local agencies, talk to members of your adoption support group, or join a group specifically for international adoptive families to find out which agency parents used.

Choosing a Country

At the time this book was written, international adoptions were mainly available from the following countries:

- Bolivia
- Bulgaria
- Cambodia
- China
- Columbia
- Guatemala
- Haiti
- India
- Mexico
- Philippines
- Romania
- Russia and former Soviet republics
- South Korea
- Thailand
- Vietnam

Each country has its own requirements. Most countries require that a couple be married for at least three years and have age limits. Russia requires that parents make two trips to the country — one to identify the child and the second to adopt him or her.

Some parents go into the adoption process knowing which country they want to adopt from, while others have no preference and choose a country that seems to fit them best. When choosing a country you will want to consider:

> **From the Expert**
>
> The *U.S. Department of State* has country-specific information available on its website. The document for each country on the site spells out the requirements and U.S. agencies that handle adoptions for that country. Visit it at:
> **http://travel.state.gov/ family/family_1732.html**

- your feelings about each country's culture and history;
- your feelings about the physical attributes common to children from that country;
- your own background and family history;
- your feeling about raising children of different ethnicity than yours;
- the type of medical care birth mothers receive in each country;
- whether or not you need to travel to that country to adopt;
- the length of stay required and the number of visits required to adopt in each country;
- the ease with which paperwork is processed in that country; and,
- the experiences of other adoptive parents who have adopted from that country.

The selection of a country is a matter of personal choice. There is not room in this book to discuss the differences between the various countries, so it is important that you do some research on your own. Start with the US Department of State website and the websites about adoption in the various countries listed in Appendix A.

Choosing a Child

In some countries, you go to the orphanage and actually select a child that appeals to you, while other countries assign a child to you. If you adopt from South Korea, you will not meet your child until he or she is delivered to you at the airport in the US.

Medical concerns are important to consider when selecting a child. Because the standard of health care varies greatly overseas, many children available for placement are developmentally delayed or suffer from a minor or major health problem. Before you choose a child, obtain photos, videotape if possible, as well as whatever medical records can be translated into English. Have them reviewed by a pediatrician who specializes in evaluating children for overseas adoptions. If you will not have access to these documents before you travel overseas, make arrangements before you leave to fax or send these items to the doctor while you are there. This kind of doctor can evaluate the child from the records and make an educated inference about what kinds of problems the child is or may be experiencing. Based on the evaluation, you may decide to adopt a different child.

> ### From the Expert
>
> The *American Academy of Pediatrics* provides a list of pediatricians specializing in adoption. View the list at:
> **www.aap.org/sections/ adoption/adopt-states/ adoption-map.html**

It is imperative that the child you select is legally released for adoption by the country of origin. Only children who are completely released for adoption will be eligible for adoption in the eyes of the US government. You will need your agency's help to obtain this release.

You have the right to turn down the child that is offered to you. Often this happens after the medical reports are examined or after you meet the child. Some parents do not wish to adopt a child with serious medical problems, while others are comfortable doing so. This is a matter of personal choice. It is important that you work with professionals you can trust who can give you good advice about medical history and developmental delays.

If you decide not to accept the child, you do not return to square one. All of the paperwork you have provided will still be valid, but you will have to wait for another child to be selected for you. The process differs in each country. You may have to return home (if you are visiting the country) or you may be able to

> **From the Expert**
> For information about how to evaluate an infant, see:
> **http://adoptingfrom russia.com/Medical Evaluation.html**

have another child assigned to you while you are there. Be sure to ask your agency how this process will work when you begin the process so there are no surprises.

Dealing with Paperwork

Your application for the adoption will be made to your local agency. They will be your primary contact throughout the entire adoption process and will handle most of the contact with the overseas agency. The application and home study process for an international adoption is similar to that required for a domestic adoption, with a few extra steps. All of these documents must be translated and then approved by the agency in the country you are adopting from (your agency will arrange for the translation). Additionally, many of the documents you provide must be authenticated, meaning they must bear a raised seal from the agency or office issuing them (there is an additional fee for obtaining authenticated copies). You may need to include photos of your home for review by the overseas agency.

In addition to the usual home study and application, you will also need to obtain preliminary USCIS approval. If you are married, one spouse must be a US citizen and your combined income must be 25% above the poverty level. You are not eligible if you have been convicted of a felony or certain misdemeanors.

The Process

Because each country has its own requirements, there is no one set procedure for international adoptions. However, the procedure you must follow in the US is the same.

You will need to complete the application, home study process (your home study will be used both by the agency as well as the USCIS to determine that you are qualified to adopt) and background check (which is also submitted to USCIS). Fingerprints must be completed at a USCIS office using the provided form FD-258. Fingerprinting will occur at your home USCIS office if you are in the U.S. or at an embassy or consulate if you are abroad.

Before you even have a child selected for adoption, you can begin the adoption process by filing form I-600A, *Orphan Petition*. It begins the process of classifying the child you will adopt as an *immediate relative*. The fee for filing is $460. You also need to file form I-864. It is an affidavit about your ability to support a child. All USCIS forms must be filed at your local office. (See Appendix B for a copy of the form.)

> **From the Expert**
> You can complete the forms online at:
> **http://uscis.gov/graphics/ formsfee/forms**

Once you have been approved to adopt by the agency and the US government, you will need to learn about the requirements for finalizing the adoption in the overseas country your child is from. This may include a court appearance in the country's court. If so, it is important that you have a translator along, which your agency can help you arrange. You may need to travel to the country and stay there for a period of time before you are permitted to adopt. You may need to appear in court in the country to finalize the adoption. Obtain several official copies of any documents you are provided by the officials you work with in the country.

Dealing with Immigration

To bring your child to the US, you must do the following.

- Use form I-600 to petition to have the identified child classified as an *immediate relative*. (If you filed form I-600A there is no fee for form I-600. If you did not, there is a $460 fee).
- Apply for the child to immigrate to the US.

You must physically see your child in person before you are permitted to adopt him or her. If a married couple is adopting, only one member of the couple must see the child in order for the adoption to be valid. If you are not adopting your child abroad and instead are only adopting him or her in the US, be sure you check that box on the *Orphan Petition*.

Visas

A *visa* is a document that gives tentative permission for the child to enter the United States from a foreign country. The visa itself is not complete authority, since immigration officials have the final say upon the child's entrance to the country.

To apply for a visa for your child, use form IR-3, for children adopted in a foreign country, or IR-4, for children that will be adopted in the US. The application must be submitted to the US embassy or consular office in the country the child is being adopted from. The child must be seen by the consular or embassy official and must also be examined by a physician approved by the consulate or embassy. Certain contagious diseases may be the basis for temporarily denying a visa. The adoptive parents must appear at the consulate or embassy for an interview. There is a $260 fee to apply for the visa and a $65 fee for the issuance of the visa.

Citizenship

Part of the adoption process is helping your child become a United States citizen. There are several ways this can occur.

Child Citizenship Act of 2000

The federal *Child Citizenship Act of 2000* allows an internationally adopted child to automatically become a US citizen. In order for the act to apply, the child must:

- have one US parent (adoptive);
- be legally adopted by this parent;
- be under age 18;

- live with the US parent that has custody of the child; and,
- be admitted to the US as an immigrant for lawful permanent residence (under an IR-4 Visa).

If these requirements are satisfied, your child will automatically be granted citizenship when the adoption is legal in the US.

To become a citizen, your child's passport (from his or her country of origin) will be stamped with USCIS Stamp I-551. You can then apply for a passport for your child (a passport will be your child's proof of citizenship). To apply for a passport, you need the following:

- DSP-11, Application for a Passport;
- two (2) identical photographs (2x2 inches in size);
- the parent's valid identification;
- certified adoption decree (with English translation, if necessary);
- the child's foreign passport with USCIS Stamp I-551 or the child's Resident Alien Card; and,
- the fee payment.

Readoption

Because United States courts are not required to legally recognize an adoption completed in a foreign country, it is a good idea to adopt your child in your state court, even if you have already completed an adoption process in the child's country of origin. At this time you will obtain a new birth certificate. This will ensure your child has an accurate birth certificate that is acceptable in the US.

Changes in Adoption Law

At the time this book was published, the US was close to approving changes to international adoption law. The *Hague Convention on*

Intercountry Adoption is an international document that provides procedures and rules for how international adoptions are handled and processed. If the US does adopt these rules, there will be some changes to the way international adoptions are handled to ensure that the children placed for adoption are truly available. Some experts say the changes will complicate the international adoption process, while others say the changes will provide important protections for all involved in the process.

From the Expert

To read more about proposed changes in how international adoptions are handled and the effects of a change, see:
http://uscis.gov/graphics/ services/HagueFS.pdf

Forms Checklist for International Adoption

❏ passports (if you will be traveling to your child)
❏ parent's birth certificate — three copies
❏ marriage certificate — three copies
❏ divorce decree (if applicable) — three copies
❏ home study
❏ fingerprints
❏ criminal background check
❏ medical reports — two copies
❏ reference letters
❏ form I-600A and/or I-600 Orphan Petition
❏ form I-864 Affidavit of Support
❏ form IR-3 or IR-4 to apply for a visa

International Agency Questionnaire

Name of Agency_____

Name of Contact Person_____

Date of Interview_____

Questions:

❑ What countries do you have agreements with?_____

❑ How many children have you placed from each of these countries in the last year?_____

❑ How long have you worked with each country?_____

❑ Do the overseas agencies you work with also work with other U.S. agencies?_____

❑ Who works overseas for your agency?_____

❑ How do babies come into the programs?_____

❑ How long will the process take?_____

❑ If parents must travel to complete the adoption, what arrangements and assistance do you provide for the trip? _____

    ❑ Is a travel agency involved?_____

    ❑ Is an escort provided?_____

    ❑ Is a translator provided?_____

    ❑ Can the agency be reached by phone outside of business hours while we are overseas?_____

❑ What access is provided to the children overseas?_____

❑ Can the agency provide referrals to Western doctors in the overseas country while we are there, should the need arise?_____

❑ Are you licensed in this state?_____

❑ How long have you been doing international adoptions?_____

❑ If a parent turns down a child, can he or she adopt another child?____

❑ What kinds of services do you provide after placement?_____

Chapter 20

Parent-Initiated Adoption

A *parent-initiated adoption* is also sometimes called a *private* or *independent adoption*. The adoptive parents locate a birth mother on their own without help from an adoption agency. The reasons for doing this are often because the couple wants to adopt a newborn, the couple does not want to work with an agency, the couple wants more control over the process, or the couple wants more in-depth contact with the birth mother than is often allowed in agency adoptions.

While a parent-initiated adoption can offer a lot of freedom, it has some drawbacks. The main concern is that if you go through the adoption process without an agency involved, you may not be completely aware of all the laws and regulations you need to comply with. Additionally, there is always the chance that the birth mother will change her mind. While this does happen with agency adoptions, the likelihood increases when an agency is not involved to counsel and support the birth mother in making this decision. An agency can often provide an experienced hand that will guide your adoption and help you get over any bumps in the road.

On the other hand, a parent-initiated adoption allows you to do things your way, without having to apply to an agency or jump through their hoops. You locate a birth mother that you feel a connection with and you handle the process yourself (with help from your attorney).

Parent-initiated adoption is not permitted in Colorado, Connecticut, Delaware, Massachusetts, and Wisconsin. In these states you must use an agency for the adoption process. However, you can still locate a birth mother on your own and then have the adoption handled by an agency.

Adopting Independently with an Agency

Many parents who choose to locate a birth mother on their own use an agency to handle the actual adoption process itself. To do so, you need to interview agencies in your area and choose one that will handle a parent-initiated adoption. The agency will coordinate the home study, provide counseling, and work with your attorney to complete the adoption process. If you are comfortable working with an agency in this way, it can make the entire process go much more smoothly. There is an intermediary between you and the birth mother and you have someone handling the paperwork on your behalf.

> ### From the Expert
> For support with and information about private adoption, contact:
> *Families for Private Adoption*
> P.O. Box 6375
> Washington, DC 20015-0375
> 202-722-0338
> **www.ffpa.org**

The agency will usually handle payment of the birth mother's expenses, so you need not pay them directly (it will be part of the costs you pay to the agency). However, you will have to pay an agency fee, which you would not pay if you handled the adoption directly with the birth mother.

How to Find a Birth Mother

There are several ways to go about finding a birth mother on your own. First, you may wish to talk to an attorney who is experienced in handling adoptions. Not only will the attorney help you understand the law and how you must go about contacting and reaching an agreement with a birth mother, but also, many experienced adoption attorneys have contact with birth mothers seeking adoptive parents for their babies. He or she may be able to help you find a birth mother.

Word of mouth is another excellent way to locate a birth mother. Tell your friends and family of your search and ask them to keep their ears open for you. Mention your search to coworkers and acquaintances. Some adoptive parents have business cards made up with their

> **From the Expert**
> Get more information about birth mother letters at:
> **www.canadaadopts.com/ registry/mistakes.shtml**

name, number, and a brief description along with words to the effect of, "We can provide a loving home for your baby. Please call us." Hand these out to friends and family and ask them to pass them along to anyone who might be interested. Give some to your gynecologist, family doctor, pastor, rabbi, and so on, if possible. Other couples create a letter to circulate to prospective birth mothers (this is often called a *Dear Birth Mother letter*) that describes you and your hopes to have a family.

Facilitator

Another option is to use an *adoption facilitator*. This is a professional who works to bring birth mothers and adoptive parents together. Facilitators are not licensed in most states and some states do not allow the use of facilitators. It is a good idea to speak with your attorney before approaching a facilitator. If you do decide to work with one, make sure you check references. Find out how many babies he or she has placed in total as well as in the last year. Make sure that you completely understand any fees

involved as well as what the fees would be if a birth mother changes her mind. Only California, Connecticut, Florida, and Iowa have laws specifically permitting payments to an adoption facilitator.

> **From the Expert**
> You can find a list of facilitators online at:
> **www.adoption.tk/ professional.htm**

The following areas do not permit the use of a facilitator:

- Alabama
- Colorado
- Delaware
- District of Columbia

- Illinois
- Kentucky
- Louisiana
- Maryland
- Massachusetts
- Michigan
- Nevada
- New Jersey
- New York
- North Carolina
- North Dakota
- Oklahoma
- Oregon
- Tennessee
- Texas
- Vermont
- Virginia
- West Virginia
- Wisconsin

Costs are usually less than private agency fees because the full range of services is not included in the contract. For example, you would need to pay for the home study, medical exams, counseling, and so on separately.

Advertising

The most popular method employed by adoptive parents to find a birth mother is advertising. You may have seen classified ads in your local paper or in national papers. The following states do not permit advertising by prospective parents:

- Alabama
- California
- Delaware
- Florida

- Georgia
- Idaho
- Kansas
- Kentucky
- Maine
- Massachusetts
- Nevada
- North Carolina
- Ohio
- Washington

If your ad starts with the letter "A," it will be near the top of all adoption ads in the paper. Since most classified ads are short, you will want to spend a lot of time polishing your ad so it contains the most information in the clearest way. Most ads make references to a loving home, financially stable couple, friendly neighborhoods, and other positive factors. Mentioning your professions can help if they are prestigious or sound comforting (such as a doctor, a lawyer, a nurse, or a teacher). The cost of the ad depends on where you place it, but normal classified ad rates usually apply if you are advertising in newspapers. National papers charge higher rates than local papers. Compare the circulation of the papers to determine what prices are best—the higher the circulation, the more people the ad will reach. Read the classifieds in your local paper to see some ads and get a feel for how you want yours to look.

> **From the Expert**
>
> For tips about wording and placing an ad, visit:
> **www.sass-works.com/ adoption/library/weekly/ UC102802a.htm**

Ads placed online are the newest way to locate a birth mother. Before you place an online ad, make sure you find out how many hits the site is receiving each month and ask for references. If you place an ad, you need to make sure your ad complies with all state laws, so be sure to consult with your attorney.

Do not underestimate the power of networking and getting the word out. Tell all your family and friends about your search for a baby and ask them to tell people they know. You might also consider creating a website that showcases your birth mother letter and has photos of you and your home.

Choosing a Birth Mother

Choosing a birth mother is a delicate process. When a birth mother contacts you, your first reaction might be to finalize things before she can change her mind. However, it is important to give yourself time and space to get to know her and to make this important decision. Make up a list of questions you want to ask a potential birth mother. You will not be able to ask her all of these questions the first time you talk, but you will have a written checklist of questions to ask as you have further conversations.

You must decide how comfortable you are with the answers to these questions. For example, if the birth mother smokes, you may wish to find someone else. If the birth mother gives you answers that conflict or that change over time, you may see a red flag. Try to get a sense of what the birth mother is like, what her life is like, and how serious she is about the adoption. You do not want to waste your time with someone who is not at all committed or who might just be trying to get money from you without fulfilling the agreement.

Write down the answers you get and discuss them with your adoption attorney. He or she will be able to guide you as to what kinds of problems to look for. It is easy to get emotionally invested too soon with a birth mother—the thought that this could be your baby can blind you to the warning signs. For this reason, it is important that you work carefully and closely with a professional who can help you see potential problems.

Contact with Birth Mother

Once you are in touch with a possible birth mother, it can be tempting to want to spend a lot of time talking to her and working things out.

However, once you have a birth mother who calls you (she should always call you — you should never make the initial call because you do not want to create extra pressure and you must be careful to stay within your state's legal requirements), you need to tell her a little about yourself, find out a little about her (such as when her due date is, how her health is, and if the birth father is in the picture at all), and then have her call your attorney.

Your attorney is not able to call her (this creates pressure and she must enter the adoption of her own free will), so you need to stress to her the importance of calling your attorney herself. Your attorney will then proceed from there and make arrangements for medical exams, counseling, and necessary paperwork. You will have many more opportunities to speak with the birth mother before either of you makes a decision about the adoption.

Payments

The average cost of a private adoption is about $13,000. The issue of payments involved in adoptions is a tricky one. It is unrealistic to expect a woman to place her child for adoption without any kind of financial assistance. However, laws about adoption payments were created to make sure that babies are not bought and sold. In most states, adoptive parents are expected to pay for the birth mother's medical expenses (this includes mental health counseling) during the course of her pregnancy. (See Chapter 9 for more information.) Payments are usually made through third parties — attorneys, facilitators, or agencies that are brought on board after the birth mother has been found.

If the birth mother has health insurance (and many do not), the expenses will be lower. The adoptive parents also handle the baby's expenses from birth. In some states, the law permits the adoptive parents to pay the birth mother's living expenses (basics like rent, utilities, food, and so on) during the last trimester of the pregnancy. Payments are usually permitted if they are *usual and customary* in the state. It is important that you check with your attorney before making any payments to the birth mother so that you are sure you are following your state's law exactly. Adoptive parents can also pay for the birth mother's attorney's fees if she employs an attorney. None of these payments are refundable if the birth mother chooses to keep the baby (except in Idaho, where they are reimbursable).

When you go to court to finalize your adoption, you will have to disclose to the court any payments you have made to the birth mother. For this reason, it is important that you remain within the allowable amounts in your state.

The following states specifically allow payment of birth mother's living expenses:

- Arizona—must be court approved over $1000;
- California—must be requested in writing by birth mother;
- Connecticut—includes maternity clothes;
- Florida;
- Idaho—payments may be made up to six weeks after the birth, not to exceed $2000 without court permission;
- Illinois;
- Indiana—payments may be made up to six weeks after the birth, not to exceed $3000;
- Iowa;
- Kansas;
- Louisiana—payments may be made up to forty-five days after the birth;
- Michigan—payments may be made up to six weeks after the birth;
- Minnesota—payments may be made up to six weeks after the birth;
- Missouri;
- Nevada;
- New Hampshire—payments may be made up to six weeks after the birth;
- New Jersey;
- New Mexico—payments may be made up to six weeks after the birth;
- North Carolina—payments may be made up to six weeks after the birth;
- North Dakota—payments may be made up to six weeks after the birth;
- Oregon;

- South Carolina—payment may be made for a reasonable period of time;
- Tennessee—payments may not be made forty-five days prior to birth or surrender or thirty days after without court approval;
- Utah;
- Vermont;
- Virginia; and,
- Wisconsin—up to $1000.

Counseling

Before you agree to anything, it is essential that the birth mother attend counseling. An initial evaluation will help reveal any negative feelings she has about the placement. Ongoing counseling will help her deal with the inevitable emotions she will face as she goes through the pregnancy and delivery and the adjustment period afterwards. Your attorney can assist the birth mother in locating a counselor experienced in adoption. You will pay for the cost of this counseling.

Counseling can also be helpful for the adoptive parents. As you wait for your baby to be born, you will also face anxiety, doubt, and fear. A counselor can help you work through the process and stay focused on the goal of adding a child to your family.

Counseling should be part of your agreement with the birth mother. It is a warning sign if a birth mother is resistant to counseling. At the very least, you must have a psychological evaluation done so that you know what you are dealing with. There are some instances in which counseling might not be necessary, but in general, it is considered necessary for all adoptions. Counseling is usually done separately for adoptive parents and birth mother, but there are some instances in which going together can be helpful, particularly if there are issues you need to work out of if you are trying to create a plan for how you will have contact after the birth.

> ### From the Expert
> For referrals to counselors, visit the *American Psychological Association* at:
> **www.apa.org**

If your birth mother lives in your area, you can provide her a with a list of counselors and even offer to drive her there. If she lives far away from you, you can still put together a list of counselors in her area.

Waiting for Your Child to be Born

When you use parent-initiated adoption, you are more closely in tune with what is happening with the birth mother as the pregnancy develops and you may have the opportunity to see or speak to her throughout the pregnancy. This relationship may be very close or not close at all. Each adoption is different and you will have to work within your comfort zone as well as that of the birth mother. Your attorney or adoption agency can be helpful intermediaries in this situation and can help communicate some basic rules for contact.

Some birth mothers and adoptive parents make arrangements for the adoptive parents to be present at the birth. You will need to work this out with your birth mother in advance. If you are present at the hospital, you will want to make sure the staff is aware you are the adoptive parents so that you can have access to the birth mother and baby. The birth mother will need to give her specific consent to this since the baby belongs to her until the placement occurs. If she does not consent, you have no right to see her or the baby.

Paperwork

As with any other adoption, the adoption is not finalized and complete until the waiting period is up, which varies depending on the state the child is born in. (See Chapter 16 for more information.) Any agreements you make with the birth mother before this are all subject to revocation of her consent to the adoption. While you and the birth mother will sign documents (that will vary by state) indicating that you consent to the adoption, this can all change if the birth mother changes her mind within the revocation period.

It is essential that you use an attorney to draft all the adoption documents. You will want to be sure that the papers you and the birth mother sign and present to the court are correct for your state and legally acceptable to the court. The birth mother must have her own attorney and cannot use yours. The court may scrutinize a parent-initiated adoption more closely than an agency adoption to be sure that state laws about payment and consent have been carefully followed.

NOTE: *If you and the birth mother live in different states, you will need to hire an attorney to represent you in each state. First choose an attorney in your home state. He or she will be able to locate an attorney in the other state to assist with the case.*

Once the waiting period concludes, the adoption is legalized and you become parents. (See Chapter 16 for more information about adoption paperwork and about birth certificates.)

Adjustment Period

After the adoption has been finalized in your state, the legal process is over for you, but the adjustment process will probably still continue. You will need to find a way to manage contact with the birth mother. Hopefully this was something you discussed and worked out with her while you were waiting for the birth, but do not be surprised if things do not go as planned. Some birth mothers who wanted regular contact may find it is less painful to get some distance and move on with their lives. Other birth mothers who thought they would want little contact may find they want more than originally thought.

Keep in mind that you are now the legal parent of this child and you are the one making the decisions. It is a good idea to try to be fair to the birth mother simply because this is what is right to do for your child, but you must make the ultimate decision about what is best for your child and what works for your family.

Choosing a Facilitator
Questionnaire

Name of Facilitator_____

Date of Interview_____

Questions:

❏ How many adoptions have you placed in the last year?_____

_____

❏ Can you provide references?_____

_____

❏ How long have you been doing this?_____

_____

❏ How many clients do you work with each year?_____

_____

❏ How do you find birth mothers?_____

_____

❏ How do you evaluate birth mothers?_____

_____

❏ What is your success rate?_____

_____

❏ How many of your birth mothers change their minds?_____

_____

❏ What are your fees?_____

_____

Potential Birth Mother Questionnaire

Name of Birth Mother_____

Date of Interview_____

Questions:

❏ Why are you placing this child for adoption?_____
_____

❏ How far along are you?_____
_____

❏ What is your due date?_____
_____

❏ Who knows about your pregnancy?_____
_____

❏ Who is the birth father?_____
_____

❏ Is he aware of the pregnancy?_____
_____

❏ Have you seen a doctor?_____
_____

❏ Who is your doctor?_____
_____

❏ Do you have any medical conditions?_____
_____

❏ Do you want an open adoption and if so, what do you mean by that term?_____
_____

❏ What are you looking for in the adoptive parents?_____
_____

❏ Do you have a job?_____
_____

❏ What do you do?_____
_____

continued

❏ Do you smoke, drink, or take any medication?_____

❏ Are you taking prenatal vitamins?_____

❏ What is your family medical history?_____

❏ What is your ethnic heritage?_____

❏ How old are you?_____

❏ What education do you have?_____

❏ Where do you live?_____

❏ Who do you live with?_____

❏ Are you in a relationship?_____

❏ Do you have other children?_____

❏ Have you placed any other children for adoption?_____

❏ Have you talked with a counselor or adoption agency about placement?

❏ What kind of support system do you have in place?_____

❏ Can you provide photos of yourself and other family members? _____

❏ How long have you known about the pregnancy?_____

Chapter 21

Single-Parent Adoption

Single-parent adoption is more commonplace than it ever used to be. Every state now recognizes that a good home does not depend on having two parents present and allows adoption by singles.

Considerations for Single-Parent Adoption

When you seek to adopt as a single, the primary concern that agencies and social workers will have is that you have a support system in place. Before seeking to adopt, give some thought to who will help you; who can provide child care; and, how you will provide role models of both sexes for your child. Family and friends provide excellent backup as well as opposite-sex role models.

When making the decision to adopt as a single person, it is important to realize the weight of the decision. A child will be completely dependent on you. You also will carry the financial and emotional burden alone—as well as deal with all of the logistics of raising the child.

Before you adopt, it is important to carefully think through all the possible scenarios—how your child will be cared for while you work; how you will afford the additional expenses; who you will turn to for help; how you will continue to have a social life; who will care for your child should you die; and, so on.

Bias Against Single Parents

While single-parent adoption is permitted in all states, some agencies and social workers continue to hold a bias against prospective single adoptive parents. If you encounter this kind of bias, it is best to confront it head-on and provide a lot of information for the agency or worker about your support system and deal with their concerns up front. There is often particular bias against single men seeking to adopt, based on misguided suspicions about pedophilia. Single men may have to work harder to convince agencies and social workers about their reasons for wanting to adopt, but have the same rights to adopt as anyone else. No one can turn you down for adoption simply because you are not married; however, other excuses may be used to discourage you. If you are confronting bias, it is a signal that you need to seek out another less judgmental agency.

There is also often an assumption that a single seeking to adopt must be gay. (See Chapter 22 for information about gay and lesbian adoption.) While you may be asked about your sexual orientation as part of the home study process, it should not matter what your orientation is as long as you have a lifestyle that is conducive to parenting.

> **From the Expert**
>
> For information and support, contact:
> *National Council for Single Adoptive Parents*
> P.O. Box 55
> Wharton, NJ 07885
> **www.adopting.org/ncsap.html**

Home Studies

You may need to work a little harder than married couples to get through the home study. You will need to show the social worker that you have thought through all the possibilities and have come up with a plan or with solutions to deal with them. Generally, it will be important to demonstrate a support network of family and friends who can step in to help. You should show that you have given thought to child care and that you know how to arrange your finances so that you can handle the extra expenses. You should also create a plan to take some time off when the adoption happens so you can bond with your child and ease the adjustment. Make it clear that you have planned this very well and that you feel secure in your ability to handle it. You will also need to show that you have a plan in place so that others are available to care for your child should you become ill, tied up at work, or have to go out of town. You should also mention that you plan to have a will drawn up that will name a guardian for your child.

Laws Governing Single-Parent Adoption
All states permit singles to adopt. However, there are a few catches. In Utah, where adoption by singles is permitted, anyone who is unmarried and cohabiting is not permitted to adopt. Florida and Mississippi do not permit adoption by anyone who is homosexual. Korea is currently the one foreign country that does not permit adoption of its children by singles.

Protecting Your Family
Single parents who adopt should consider purchasing disability insurance and life insurance to provide for their family's financial security. It will also be essential to execute a will naming a guardian for your child. You may wish to execute this will before your adoption is finalized. (There has been a case in which a woman had a fatal accident as she was returning home with her newly adopted child and since she had no will, the court had to decide on a guardian.)

Raising Your Child
With more and more people divorcing and singles adopting or having children without a partner, the single-parent family is no longer an oddity. Few people will give your adoption a second thought. However, there are some people who will simply not understand that your child does not have another parent. They will assume you must be divorced or not living with your child's other parent.

As you raise your child, you will encounter some bumps in the road. There is just one of you and you cannot be in all places at all times.

Conflicts will come up, but if you have a support network in place, your child will be well cared for. Make sure that you leave room in your life for friends and for dating, if that is what you are interested in. You may be a parent, but you are still a person. You should be able to continue to work hard at your career, have fun, and spend some money on yourself. Parenting is not all about sacrifice.

Realize that although single parenting is easy for you to accept, it may not be easy for other people to accept. You may find yourself explaining more times than you wish that no your child does not have another parent and no, you are not widowed or divorced. As your child grows, spend some time explaining the different kinds of families and how you came to be a single parent.

Children of single-parent families thrive and do just as well as children from families with two parents. In short, adopting a child on your own does not provide any particular roadblocks or problems for your child, unless you create them.

Gay and Lesbian Adoption

In recent years, the laws about same-sex couple adoption have become more encompassing as more and more states have accepted gay couples as adoptive parents. There are several paths to consider when you and your partner want to become parents.

Single-Parent Adoption

If you are gay and single, your sexual orientation should not come into play with adoption. The information contained in Chapter 16 details the process and procedures you should follow. However, the information contained in this chapter will provide some specific information for a gay or lesbian person seeking to adopt.

Second-Parent Adoption

If one partner has a child (that is his or her natural child or is a child he or she adopted) and the other partner would like to adopt the child, a second-parent adoption procedure can be used. (See Chapter 17 for more information about second-parent adoptions.) There are some restrictions on same-sex, second-parent adoption, since it is not permitted in all states.

The areas that permit same-sex, second-parent adoption include:

- California
- Connecticut
- District of Columbia

- Illinois
- Massachusetts
- New Jersey
- New York
- Vermont

Other states have permitted some same-sex, second-parent adoptions, but do not have a clear-cut policy. These states include:
- Alabama
- Alaska
- Delaware
- Georgia
- Hawaii
- Indiana
- Iowa
- Louisiana
- Maryland
- Michigan
- Minnesota
- Nevada
- New Mexico
- Oregon
- Rhode Island
- Texas
- Washington

Florida completely disallows adoption by gays, as does Mississippi. Utah law does not allow unmarried people who are cohabiting to adopt.

Although the laws that permit second-parent adoption treat it as a separate process, in reality, gay couples are really adopting together. Yes, one partner must be the one to initially adopt the child and then the other partner can do a second-parent adoption, but these are just legal terms and processes and you should not get too bogged down with them. You are adopting together and you will parent together. There is no reason to think of it in any other way. (The American Academy of Pediatrics formally supports second-parent adoption by gay partners.)

Couple Adoption

Gay couples can adopt a child together, simultaneously, in Washington D.C., New York, New Jersey, Vermont, and California. Most other states have laws that are not clear on this issue.

> **From the Expert**
> Read your state adoption laws at:
> **www.lambdalegal.org**
> or
> **http://straylight.law. cornell.edu/topics/Table_ Adoption.htm**

However, this does not mean gay couples cannot adopt in most states. The best procedure to use in other states is a two-step adoption. In the first step, one partner adopts the child alone. He or she can use an agency or independent adoption — whatever method works best for him or her. Once that adoption is complete, then the other partner can seek a second-parent adoption of the child in those states that permit second-parent adoptions by gay partners.

International Adoption

Gay adoption is not permitted by any international country. However, this does not mean a gay single or couple cannot adopt. Single-parent international adoption is possible if you are not open about your sexuality. If you are a couple, the child can then be adopted by the other parent via a second-parent adoption procedure.

> **From the Expert**
> For a list of countries with policies against gay adoption, visit:
> **http://adoption.about.com/ od/gaylesbian/a/ gayadopt.htm**

Finding Gay-Friendly Adoption Agencies

To find a gay-friendly agency, talk to other same-sex couples who have adopted. Contact your local gay pride organization and ask for information about agencies they are aware of.

If you and/or your partner are seeking an agency adoption, it will be important to carefully question the agency about their policies regarding same-sex adoption. Listen not only to the official, written policy, but also to the nuances you pick up when talking to agency employees, in the literature you receive, and in all of your contacts with the agency. You want an agency that is comfortable with you and that will work to the best of its ability to place a child with you. If the birth mothers play a role in selecting adoptive parents, you will have a second barrier to deal with. Each birth mother will have her own preferences and opinions.

If the agency policy is accepting and welcoming, make sure you use one of the social workers employed by or recommended by the agency to avoid any potential bias when you go through the home study process. During the home study process it will be important to demonstrate that your relationship is solid and committed. If you have registered with any domestic partner registries, obtained a civil union or gay marriage license, or completed any affidavits for employers about your relationship (often required in order to access health benefits for a partner), it is important to share this information with your social worker. You should also mention a commitment ceremony or wedding, if you had one.

Public agencies are always a safe bet if your state has laws specifically permitting adoption by gays. There are always children available for adoption through public agencies, although they are usually not infants and may have special needs. (See Chapter 18 for more information about public agencies.)

> **From the Expert**
>
> The *Human Rights Campaign* offers a database of gay-friendly adoption agencies at:
> **www.hrc.org/Template.cfm ?Section=Adoption**
>
> Then click on "Adopting through an Agency."

Raising an Adoptive Child

Unfortunately, there is still discrimination against gays and their children. As you raise your child, you will need to be on the lookout for schools, camps, and organizations that will accept and welcome your child and your family. Keep an eye out for literature that refers to *parents* instead of *mothers* and *fathers*. Ask about gay-straight alliances (GSAs), school organizations that strive to support and include all students from all families. (The 1984 *Equal Access Law* held that if a school receives federal funds and has a limited open forum (meaning they allow other noncurriculum based groups to meet and use school resources), then the school cannot discriminate about which types of groups the school allows or supports.)

> ### From the Expert
> For information and support about gay parenting, contact:
> *Family Pride Coalition*
> P.O. Box 65327
> Washington, DC 20035-5327
> 202-331-5015
> **www.familypride.org**

As you raise your child, you will find ways to talk to your child about being gay. Remember that being gay does not mean your child will be gay. Your child will have questions about your life, but for the most part it will feel completely natural to him or her. You and your child will probably encounter discrimination and ignorance. Spending time with other gay families or helping your child find support is important.

Your child will need role models from the opposite sex. Work with other gay or lesbian families to provide this kind of support. You can also make sure your child spends time with straight family and friends so that he or she comes to know and love people of all types.

If you and your partner adopt your child together, you may encounter

> ### From the Expert
> The *Gay, Lesbian and Straight Educational Network* can provide more information about school inclusiveness. Contact them at 212-727-0135 or
> **www.glsen.org**

From the Expert

Help your child understand and deal with social reactions and help him or her understand the issues and your point of view by sharing books, such as those on the list created by *Children of Lesbians and Gays Everywhere* at:

www.colage.org/pubs/ books_for_kids.pdf

ignorance and unpleasantness at times. Many people are still unaware of the fact that gay couples can adopt children together and be legal parents together. You may have to offer proof to get someone to believe you — such as showing a birth certificate. Try to keep in mind that everything you do makes it easier for those gay couples or singles who come after you, so every bit of education or eye opening you do has meaning and purpose.

Chapter 23

Coping with Adoption

Adoption might be one of the bright moments in your life, but there will be bumps along the road as you work through the process. Working through the difficulties and disappointments might not be easy but will be worth it once you achieve your ultimate goal of adopting a child.

Dealing with Reactions to Adoption

While most people think of adoption as a good thing, there still seems to be a need to distinguish between adoptive children and biological children. Parents who adopt a child that does not resemble them will often be asked if the child is adopted. Some people go on to ask for details about the adoption. Each person who adopts has to make his or her own decision about how much information they are willing to share with other people about the adoption. You may feel that it is no one's business but yours and your child's. In fact, some adoptive parents choose not to discuss anything about the adoption with others and simply come up with an appropriate response that closes the subject for good.

Some parents decide that they are not going to discuss their child's origins with people they do not know. For instance, if you adopt a child from Korea and you are not Asian, people may come up to you and ask where your child is from, whether you knew his or her parents, and other details about the adoption. While these questions are often well-intentioned, they send a message to your child that he or she is different, that there is something strange in the way he or she entered your family, and that it is something to be questioned or discussed. Some parents choose not to discuss these details with other people and instead respond by explaining that they do not wish to discuss the private details of their family with other people.

You may also encounter people who assume that because you adopted, you had fertility problems. This is a misconception (so to speak!), since many people choose adoption without attempting to get pregnant.

What can be most disconcerting is the feeling that because you adopted your child, some people believe he or she is not really *yours* in the same way a biological child would be. People have a tendency to make a distinction between biological children and adopted children. You never hear anyone referring to someone's child as their biological child, but you quite often hear a reference to a person's adopted child. This is the kind of distinction many adoptive parents are working to change. Those who adopt know that it does not matter how a child comes to you. Your child is your child and how he or she joined your family is simply not important.

Dealing with Others Involved in Your Case

Because adoptions sometimes take longer than it seems they should, it is easy to become frustrated and annoyed with the people who seem to be holding it up—or at least not moving it along as quickly as you would like. While it is sometimes necessary to ask the tough questions and find out why there are delays, it is important to remember that you need to deal with the people involved with your adoption in a polite and friendly way. While adding a child to your family is a critical event for you, these people are simply doing their jobs—as rewarding as that may be—and they do not have the same sense of urgency, impatience, and frustration that you may feel.

While it is understandable that you may express your frustration and want solid answers about delays or problems, it is not a good idea to personally attack or argue with workers and officials. These people are the ones who are moving your case along. In general, you want to be cooperative when dealing with them and your goal should be to get them to like you if possible. Things move more quickly when there are good relations in place.

When dealing with an international adoption, it can be even more frustrating to have your fate held up by people you cannot even communicate with. When doing an international adoption, it is important that you work closely with your agency and that you are able to trust them to handle things for you. Make sure that if you travel to your child's country of origin, you know how to reach your agency at all hours if there is a problem or if you need help.

Dealing with the Waiting

Whether you are waiting through a birth mother's pregnancy, for a foreign country to match you with a child, or for a domestic agency to complete your home study, you will feel a level of anxiety and impatience. Remind yourself that adoption is a long process. Take things one step at a time and try to enjoy a sense of progress each time you move closer to the final resolution.

Joining an adoption support group can give you a place to talk about your feelings, offer you the chance to hear other people's experiences, and get advice. The waiting game can be hard on a relationship as well. You and your spouse or partner may find that you are on edge or more tense than usual. This too is normal. Remember that you are in this together and have the same ultimate goal.

Dealing with Doubts

Adoption is a life-changing event. It is normal to experience doubts or have questions about the entire decision or process. The best way to deal with doubts or questions is head-on. Look closely at your concerns. If you are doubting your ability to care for or love your adoptive child, you can rest assured that there will not be a problem once that child comes home to you. Counseling can be a big help in getting you to identify things you are worried or uncomfortable about and providing an outlet for you to

> ### From the Expert
> You can find online adoption support at:
> **http://parenting.adoption. com/parents/parenting-support-forums.html**

work through the issues. If you are worried about parenting skills, consider taking a parenting class.

Doubts about the agency, birth mother, or social worker should be carefully considered. Express your concerns to the agency or to your attorney. Try to talk through these concerns and obtain reassurances to ease your mind. That being said, there are times when you just know something is wrong or not working. In those instances you should listen to your gut feelings.

Changing Your Mind

You can change your mind about the adoption any time until it is finalized. You may still be liable for expenses and fees up to that point. If you have serious unresolved doubts about the adoption or your situation has changed so that adoption is no longer a good decision for you, it is better to confront them now before you become an adoptive child's parent. The child you were going to adopt will be placed elsewhere, so you need not feel guilty.

Some families are lucky enough to unexpectedly become pregnant while attempting to adopt a child. The pregnancy does not affect your ability to adopt, unless *you* decide that it does.

Taking Time Off for Your Adoption

You should check with your employer to determine if they offer time off to complete an adoption. Some employers have special provisions for this in order to encourage and support adoption. You can also plan to take time off once the adoption is complete under the federal *Family and Medical Leave Act* (FMLA) or your state family leave law (check with your human resources department to determine if your state has such a law). You are eligible for a federal FMLA leave if you work for a public agency (federal, state or local) or for a private employer with fifty or more employees and have been employed there at least twelve months and worked at least 1250 hours in the last twelve months. You can take up to twelve weeks of unpaid leave and you can take this time all together or break it up, or even use it to return to work part-time after the adoption. When possible, you must provide your employer with thirty days notice, but in some adoption cases this is not possible.

> ### From the Expert
> If you experience any problems with your FMLA request, contact the *Department of Labor* at:
> **www.dol.gov**

Under FMLA, your employer must keep your health benefits in place (but you may have to pay premiums while you are out) and must restore you to original job or to an equivalent job with equivalent pay when you return. Your employer cannot penalize you for taking the leave or allow it to affect any of your benefits. If you return to work and your employer has taken away some of your job responsibilities or cut your hours, this would be a violation.

If you and your spouse work for the same employer, you are entitled to a total of twelve weeks unpaid FMLA leave divided between both of you in a twelve-month period to care for your child. So for example, you could take ten weeks and your spouse could take two weeks. Your leaves can be taken simultaneously. Spouses who work for different employers are entitled to each take the full FMLA twelve weeks.

Bonding with an Adopted Child

Many adoptive parents are worried about how well they will bond with their child. When a child becomes part of your life, your heart will open to make room for him or her. There is often the expectation that bonding is immediate—that once you see or hold your child you will immediately fall in love with him or her. Sometimes bonding is a gradual process, so do not be disappointed or upset if it takes you a little while to adjust to the new person in your life.

> ### From the Expert
> Read about attachment and bonding issues at:
> **http://attachment. adoption.com/index.php**

Dealing with Adoption Disappointments

Occasionally adoption disappointments happen—a birth mother might decide not to place her newborn, a child that has been selected for you might have needs you feel you cannot meet, or something else may go wrong during the process to keep an adoption from happening. Birth mothers have the right to change their minds after the birth, so no adoption is certain until the court has made it legal. If you do experience a disappointment like this, it is important to give yourself time and room to deal with it. A particular dream that you had has ended. Some potential adoptive parents decide that they cannot try to adopt again after a disappointment, but most do try again. You might need some time or you might be able to move forward immediately to find a new child or birth mother.

From the Expert

Support and assistance with failed adoptions is available at:

http://forums.adoption.com/ f410.html

Adoption support groups can be a lifesaver when you are confronted with a disappointment, so seek one out if you need support or advice.

Chapter 24

Raising an Adopted Child

Once an adoption is complete, you can move on to the joy of being a family and raising your new child. However, raising an adopted child is not always the same as raising a biological child and there are some concerns and issues that may arise.

Celebrating Your Adoption

Once your adoption is complete, you will probably want to introduce your new family member to friends and family. Some people choose to send adoption announcements or hold a celebration or ceremony to welcome the child into the family. Many families treat an adoption as they would any other birth, with a baby shower.

As your child grows, you will need to think about how you will recognize the adoption. Some families hang special plaques in their home to commemorate an adoption. Other families celebrate their child's adoption day each year with a special celebration. Each family must make its own decisions about what they are comfortable with and what is the best way to mark this important event.

Breastfeeding an Adopted Infant

It is possible to breastfeed an adopted infant. Some mothers choose to breastfeed an adopted infant because of the known health benefits of breastfeeding or as a way to bond with the child, provide comfort, and

From the Expert

For more information on breastfeeding for adoptive parents, contact the *La Leche League* at:
www.laleche.org

The *Adoptive Breastfeeding Resource* website at:
www.fourfriends.com/abrw

create a physical connection to a child that you are not biologically connected to. For some women, it just feels natural to want to feed and nurture your child yourself.

The stimulation of nursing will cause a rise in prolactin, a hormone that stimulates milk production. However, adoptive mothers usually cannot produce enough milk on their own. Lactation aids can be used, providing supplementary formula to the infant while breastfeeding. Contact your pediatrician's office and ask to meet with a lactation consultant on staff. If your doctor is not supportive, find one who is.

Talking to Your Biological Children about Adoption

If you have biological children, the adoption of a new brother or sister will be a time of excitement as well as anxiety. Many of the concerns and problems that arise are the same as those that occur when a child is added to the family through biological means. However, there are some concerns that are unique to the adoption situation. Young children may be terrified at the thought of a parent placing a child for adoption and may fear that this will happen to them. You will need to reassure your child that you are not placing any of your children for adoption and that this happens only in very unique circumstances.

Depending on the age of your biological children, there are different ways to discuss adoption. Getting a book about adoption can be one good way to explain it to your child. Another idea is to talk to you child about all the things parents do for their children—putting them to bed, changing diapers, feeding them, loving them, and so on. Then explain to your child that another thing parents do is bring the child into the world. Explain that children who are adopted have one set of parents who bring them into the world, but are unable to do all the other things a parent has to do, so the child gets adoptive parents who will do everything else for them for the rest of their lives. This will help prevent your biological child from worrying that you will one day not want him or her and place him or her for adoption.

It is important to make sure your child does not think of an adoptive child as one who was not wanted. Focus the discussion on the birth parents not being able to care for the child and give him or her everything he or she needs. If you refer to the adopted child as unwanted, you are setting the stage for your biological child to taunt your adoptive child.

Existing children may resent the attention an adopted child receives, especially if he or she has special needs or a situation that requires a lot of time and energy from the parents. It always takes work to help everyone adjust when you add a child to the family. Adoption situations are no different. Time, patience, and understanding are often the best remedies.

Raising Biological and Adopted Siblings

If you are raising a family created through birth and adoption, there is sure to be conflict—but there is conflict any time you have siblings, whether they are biologically related or not. It is essential you treat all of your children fairly and with respect and that they understand they are all equally part of the family. It is important to emphasize to children that all people are different and family members are different too. Your differences are what make your family special. Biological children take their cues from the parents. If you feel your adopted child is a full member of your family, they will as well.

If you are raising a child of a different ethnicity or from a different culture, you may wish to educate your adoptive child and any biological children (as well as yourself) about the history, culture, and traditions of the country or group of people. Doing so gives your adopted child a sense of identity; involves your family in his or her past; and, shows that you celebrate and appreciate who your child is and where he or she came from. You may also wish to spend time with families that have adopted children with similar backgrounds. (See Appendix A for a list of such organizations.)

Talking to Your Child about His or Her Adoption

Many parents tell their child basic information about his or her adoption from the very beginning. The story of how the child joined the family becomes a treasured story that is told over and over. When talking about adoption, most experts recommend that you emphasize that the birth mother or father made the placement decision out of love and concern. Some adoptive parents choose to emphasize that the child was meant to be part of this family, while de-emphasizing the idea that another family or mother did not want the child.

It is also helpful to point out that families are made in many ways— through birth, stepparenting, surrogacy, foster care, and so on. How the family was created is unimportant, but the fact that it exists is the primary fact. When you talk to your child about adoption, be sure to share how you felt and how important the adoption was to you and the entire family. Share details of the adoption, just as you would share details of a biological child's birth.

As your child grows older, you may be able to share more details about the adoption, such as the birth mother's name or facts about her. Being open with your child about the facts will help him or her feel comfortable with his or her own personal history.

> ### From the Expert
>
> For more information about talking to your child about adoption, see:
> **www.adopting.org/talk.html**
> **www.rainbowkids.com**
> **www.adoption**
> **connection.org**

As children become older, they want and need more details and often want to know specifics about their birth parents. As an adoptive parent, your role is to supply what information you can and offer support. If you have remained in contact with the birth parent, you will have a lot you can share. If you have no identifying information about the birth parents, your child can register with various adoptee groups to attempt to make contact with the birth parents. (See Appendix A for more information.)

The amount of information you share with your child at various points in his or her life will be up to you. In large part you should take your cues from your child. Offer information when he or she is interested in learning more.

Keeping an Adoption a Secret

It is possible to keep an adoption a secret — after all, this is how adoptions used to be done. For the most part, it is not thought by experts to be a good idea anymore. Adopted children who are raised as if they are biological children may find out at some point that they were adopted. Discovering this kind of information can be very hurtful and disappointing. Think carefully about your reasons for wanting to keep the adoption a secret and how it can benefit your family. Weigh this against your child's need to know his or her own history and the sense of betrayal that is possible should the information ever be revealed.

Cultural Heritage

If your child has a cultural or ethnic heritage different than your own, you will want to share your own history and traditions with him or her. You may also want to try to incorporate some of his or her background into your family. Some adoptive parents who adopt internationally take many photos when they visit their child's country so they can later show him or her what it is like. Buying books and traditional clothing and games from your child's country is another way to help him or her connect with the past. Learn about the holidays and traditions from your child's country or ethnic group and celebrate them.

> **From the Expert**
> Consider joining an adoption support group for parents of children from specific countries such as *Families With Children From China* at:
> **www.fwcc.org/welcome.html**
>
> or *Families with Children from Vietnam* at:
> **www.fcvn.org**

Your heritage will be important to your child as well and will become part of his or her own heritage. Your child will grow up eating your family's foods and celebrating your holidays. These things will belong to him or her just as they belong to you. However, some adoptive children may at some point feel as if participating in these things is somehow false for them. With a little encouragement and enthusiasm, you can let your child know that he or she is a very real part of your cultural line.

Medical Issues

When you adopt your child, you will receive some kind of medical history for him or her. This will include information about his or her health and may include a family history if available. It is important to obtain as much information as you can. This may mean asking several times or paying for translations of documents from another language if your adoption is an international one. The more information you are able to gather, the better. While your child may come to you in good health, he or she will need a detailed history later in life and any information you can obtain will be helpful. Some children come to adoption with very little medical history. Your child still has every chance to grow up to be healthy.

Postadoption Support

Adoption support groups are great ways to get information and support while you are in the adoption process, but they are also important in the postadoption period. A support group can help you and your child through the adjustments you face right after an adoption, as well as with the ongoing issues that pop up from time to time in an adopted child's life. Children can connect with other adopted children through these groups. Also, once you have gone through an adoption, you are in the perfect position to offer help and encouragement to potential adoptive parents who contact the group for information. (See Appendix A for information on support groups.)

Finding Birth Parents

As your child matures, he or she may wish to learn more about his or her birth parents, country of origin, or background. Some parents keep scrapbooks for their adopted children that includes the birth mother letter they wrote, photos they took in the child's country of origin, photos of birth parents, adoption paperwork, or letters from birth parents. Depending on the type of adoption, finding your child's birth parent can vary in difficulty. Start with the agency you worked with and contact information you had at the time of adoption. You may need to hire an investigator to eventually find the birth parents.

Epilogue

This book has presented you with a wide variety of choices and options for building a family. You may feel more comfortable with some options than with others. You may also start down one path and later decide to follow another. There are no right or wrong choices—there are only those that work for you. As you face new decisions or challenges, this book can help you work through the choices and problems you face.

My hope is that this book helps you find the child of your heart.

Glossary

A

adoptee. Person being adopted.

adoption. A process whereby a child becomes part of another's family through legal means.

adoption assistance agreement. A contract between adoptive parents and state agency that placed the child, describing the monthly payments the state will make to the parents to help with the expense of raising a child.

adult adoption. Adoption by one adult of another adult.

agency adoption. An adoption in which an agency connects the birth mother and intended parents and handles the mechanics and paperwork.

American Association of Tissue Banks (AATB). A voluntary organization that accredits sperm and egg donation banks.

assisted reproductive treatment (ART). This is the medical assistance you receive as you try to conceive.

B

biological parent. A person who provided genetic material to create a child.

birth father. The biological father of the child.

birth mother. The biological mother of the child. Also sometimes defined as the woman who physically gave birth to the child.

birth parent. The biological parent of the child.

blastocyst. An early embryo.

C

Child Citizenship Act of 2000. A federal law that allows an internationally adopted child to automatically become a US citizen.

cloning. Different procedures used to create a copy of a cell.

closed adoption. An adoption whereby the child has no information about the birth parents.

consent. A legal agreement that an adoption should take place.

consulate. A government's office in another country, through which it can assist citizens visiting the foreign country.

cryopreservation. The freezing of eggs, sperm, or embryos.

cytoplasm. Material that fills the egg and gives it energy.

cytoplasmic transfer. A technique that removes cytoplasm from a donor egg and injects it into the mother's egg.

D

domestic adoption. An adoption of a child born in the United States.

donor. A person who donates egg, sperm, or embryo for another to use.

E

embassy. An official headquarters of a government inside a foreign country.

embryo. An egg fertilized with sperm that has begun to divide.

embryo adoption. A process in which an embryo is donated to another couple or person and adoption-type procedures are followed, such as home studies and possible contact between the parties.

embryo donation. A donation to another couple or for use in research of an embryo created during ART.

F

facilitator. A professional who arranges adoptions.

Family and Medical Leave Act **(FMLA).** A federal law that allows up to twelve weeks of unpaid time off from work when you are dealing with your own medical conditions (such as fertility treatments) or caring for a family member, such as a newborn or adopted child.

foster care. A situation in which a child that is in the custody of the state is temporarily cared for by adults licensed by the state.

foster parent. An adult who contracts with an agency to care for children who are in the custody of the state.

G

gamete. An egg or sperm cell.

gamete intrafallopian transfer (GIFT). A technique in which eggs are placed into the intended mother's fallopian tubes with large numbers of sperm.

gestational surrogacy. The intended mother's egg is implanted into the surrogate with the intended father's sperm to conceive a child. The surrogate has no biological relationship with the child.

guardianship. A legal proceeding giving someone the authority to make decisions for another person, usually a child or a person who is mentally incompetent.

H

Health Insurance Portability and Accountability Act (HIPAA). A federal law that makes medical record confidential.

home study. A process through which a licensed social worker meets with prospective adoptive parents and evaluates their lifestyle and home for its appropriateness to house a child.

I

Immigration and Naturalization Service (INS). The previous name of the department whose duties are now administered by the USCIS.

independent adoption. An adoption in which the adoptive parent locates the child or birth mother instead of having an agency do so.

Indian Child Welfare Act. A federal law specifying that a Native American child must be placed with relatives, within the tribe, or with other Native Americans before other options are considered.

informed consent. Agreeing to treatment after being apprise of all the risks and benefits. Informed consent is required before any medical procedure can be done.

induced cycle. Ovulation that is induced by medication.

insemination. A process of inserting sperm into a woman's body or into eggs in a laboratory to achieve conception.

international adoption. An adoption of a child born in another country.

intracytoplasmic sperm injection (ICSI). An injection into an egg of a single sperm, also called *microinsemination*.

in vitro fertilization (IVF). When an egg is fertilized with sperm in a laboratory.

in vitro maturation. A process that allows eggs to mature in a lab instead of inside a woman.

intrauterine insemination (IUI). A superovualtion is induced and a large number of sperm is inserted into the uterus.

K

kinship adoption. An adoption of a child that is a relative.

kinship agreement. An agreement outlining contact that birth parents and other relatives will have with a child that has been adopted.

L

legal parent. A parent who is considered to be a child's parent in the eyes of the law.

legal risk placement. A placement of a foster care child who may need to be reunited with his or her parents.

M

minor. A child under the age of eighteen.

mitrochondrial genes. Specific genes that do not determine physical traits, but can carry inherited diseases.

Multiethnic Placement Act. A federal law that denies funding to adoption agencies that delay or deny placement because of race.

N

natural cycle. Ovulation that occurs without medication or medical intervention.

notice. A legal notification of an adoption proceeding.

nuclear transfer. A process in which the nucleus of an egg cell is removed and replaced with another nucleus.

nucleus. Part of a cell that contains genetic material.

O

oocyte. An egg cell.

open adoption. An adoption in which the child is aware that he or she was adopted and one in which he or she may or may not have contact with the birth parents.

ovum. Egg cell, female reproductive cell.

P

parent-initiated adoption. An adoption in which the adoptive parent locates the child or birth mother instead of having an agency do so.

petition. A legal document asking a court to approve an adoption.

private adoption. An adoption that does not involve an agency. The birth mother and intended parents work directly with each other.

putative father registry. A state registry that allows a man to record the fact that he believes he is the father of the child, before the child is born.

R

readoption. Legal process in which parents of a child adopted internationally go through a US adoption.

revocation. Legally taking back your consent for an adoption.

S

second-parent adoption. An adoption of a child by his or her stepparent.

social worker. A professional who performs home studies and assists families with adjustments to adoptions.

somatic nuclear cloning. Replacing the nucleus of a cell with a cell from another person.

special needs child. A child that has a physical or mental disability.

sperm. Male reproductive cell.

sperm donor. Male who donates sperm to be used by a woman or couple to conceive a baby. Sperm donors can be anonymous or known.

success rate. The percent or successful pregnancies a clinic produces.

surrogacy. The process by which a surrogate carries a pregnancy for the intended parent(s) and has no legal ties to the child.

surrogacy agreement. A contract made with a surrogate in which she agrees to carry the couple's child and allow them to become the child's legal parents. It often includes provisions for the intended parents to pay her expenses through the pregnancy.

surrogate. A woman who carried a pregnancy for the intended parent(s) without any legal ties to the child.

T

take home babies. The percent or number of children conceived through ART that are born and go home with their parents. This rate is usually the most accurate way to evaluate a clinic since it does not count failed pregnancies.

traditional surrogacy. The surrogate's own eggs are used in conjunction with sperm from the intended father to conceive a child. The surrogate is biologically related to the resulting child.

U

United States Citizenship and Immigration Services (USCIS). A division of the Department of Homeland Security.

V

visa. An immigration document that allows you to enter a country.

Z

zygote intrafallopian transfer (ZIFT). A process where eggs are inseminated, then placed in the fallopian tubes.

zygote. An early embryo.

Appendix A

Resources

This appendix provides numerous additional resources as you go through the process of building a family and dealing with the issues these decisions bring. In it you will find information on books, both for adults and children, organizations, and websites all designed to help your process be more informed and supported.

Books for Adults

Infertility Titles

Alternative Beginnings:
A Woman's Guide to Getting
Pregnant by Self-Insemination
by Lisa Saffron

Choosing Assisted Reproduction:
Social, Emotional & Ethical
Considerations
by Susan Cooper

Choosing to Be Open
about Donor Conception
by Sharon Pettle and Ian Burns

Having a Baby Without a Man:
The Woman's Guide To
Alternative Insemination
by Susan Robinson, M.D. and
H.F. Pizer, P.A.C.

Helping the Stork:
The Choices and Challenges
of Donor Insemination
by Carol Frost Vercollone, et al.

The Long-Awaited Stork:
A Guide to Parenting
After Infertility
by Ellen Sarasohn Glazer

Taking Charge of Infertility
by Patricia Irwin Johnston

Adoption Titles

Adopting After Infertility
by Patricia Irwin Johnston

Adoption is a Family Affair!
What Relatives and Friends
Must Know
by Patricia Irwin Johnston

Adopting On Your Own:
The Complete Guide to Adoption
for Single Parents
by Lee Varon

Adoption Lifebook:
A Bridge to Your Child's Beginnings
by Cindy Probst

Breastfeeding the Adopted Baby
by Debra Stewart Peterson

How to Adopt Internationally:
A Guide for Agency-Directed and
Independent Adoptions
by Jean Nelson Erichsen and
Heino R. Erichsen

Is Adoption for You?:
The Information You Need
to Make the Right Choice
by Christine Adamec

Launching a Baby's Adoption:
Practical Strategies for Parents
and Professionals
by Patricia Irwin Johnston

Open Adoption Experience:
Complete Guide for Adoptive
and Birth Families
by Lois Ruskai Melina

Single Mothers by Choice:
A Guidebook for Single Women
Who Are Considering or
Have Chosen Motherhood
by Jane Mattes

Surrogate Motherhood:
Conception in the Heart
by Helena Ragone

Toddler Adoption:
The Weaver's Craft
by Mary Hopkins Best

Twenty Things Adopted Kids Wish
Their Adoptive Parents Knew
by Sherrie Eldridge

Books for Children

Infertility Titles

How Babies and Families Are
Made: There Is More Than
One Way!
by Patricia Shaffer

How I Began:
The Story of Donor Insemination
by Julia Paul

Let Me Explain:
A Story About Donor
Insemination
by Jane Schnitter

Mommy Did I Grow in Your
Tummy? Where Some Babies
Come From
by Elaine R. Gordon

Phoebe's Family:
A Story about Egg Donation
by Linda Stamm

Adoption Titles

Adoption Is for Always
by Linda Walvoord Girard

The Best Single Mom in the
World: How I Was Adopted
by Mary Zisk

The Day We Met You
by Phoebe Koehler

Did My First Mother Love Me?
A Story for an Adopted Child
by Kathryn Ann Miller

Filling in the Blanks:
A Guided Look at
Growing Up Adopted
by Susan Gabel

Happy Adoption Day!
by John McCutcheon

Heart of Mine: A Story of
Adoption
by Dan Hojer

How I Was Adopted
by Joanna Cole

I Love You Like Crazy Cakes
by Rose A. Lewis

Let's Talk About It: Adoption
by Fred Rogers

Mommy Far, Mommy Near:
An Adoption Story
by Carol Antoinette Peacock

My Special Family:
A Children's Book About
Open Adoption
by Kathleen Silber

Never Never Never
Will She Stop Loving You
by Jolene Durrant

Over the Moon: An Adoption Tale
by Karen Katz

Rosie's Family:
An Adoption Story
by Lori Rosove

Seeds of Love:
For Brothers and Sisters
of International Adoption
by Mary Ebejer Petertyl

Two Birthdays for Beth
by Gay Lynn Cronin

We Wanted You
by Liz Rosenberg

When You Were Born in China:
A Memory Book for Children
Adopted from China
by Sara Dorow

When You Were Born in Korea
by Brian E. Boyd

Where Are My Birth Parents?:
A Guide for Teenage Adoptees
by Karen Gravelle

Who Am I?:
And Other Questions of Adopted
Kids (Plugged in)
by Charlene C. Giannetti

Why Was I Adopted?
by Carole Livingston

Magazines

Infertility Titles

Conceive Magazine
7512 Doctor Phillips Boulevard
Suite 50, PMB 205
Orlando, FL 32819
800-758-0770
www.conceivemagazine.com

Adoption Titles

Adoption TODAY Magazine
541 East Garden Drive, Unit N
Windsor, CO 80550
888-924-6736
www.adoptinfo.net

Adoptive Families Magazine
42 West 38th Street
Suite 901
New York, NY 10018
646-366-0830
www.adoptivefamilies.com

Adopting for Tomorrow
5165 West Woodmill Drive
Suite 12
Wilmington, DE 19808
888-281-1284
www.adoptingtomorrow.com

Organizations

Infertility

American Infertility Association
666 Fifth Avenue
Suite 278
New York, NY 10103
888-917-3777
www.theafa.org

*American Society for
Reproductive Medicine*
1209 Montgomery Highway
Birmingham, Alabama 35216-2809
205-978-5000
www.asrm.org

Family Pride Coalition
P.O. Box 65327
Washington, DC 20035
202-231-5015
www.familypride.org

*The International Council on Infertility
Information Dissemination, Inc.*
P.O. Box 6836
Arlington, VA 22206
703-379-9178
www.inciid.org

*OPTS Organization of Parents
Through Surrogacy*
P.O. Box 611
Gurnee, IL 60031
847-782-0224
www.opts.com

*RESOLVE
The National Infertility Association*
1310 Broadway
Somerville, MA 02144
888-623-0744
www.resolve.org

Snowflakes
Nightlight Christian Adoptions
801 East Chapman
Suite 106
Fullerton, CA 92831
714-278-1020
www.snowflakes.org

Adoption

American Academy of
Adoption Attorneys
P.O. Box 33053
Washington, DC 20033
202-832-2222
www.adoptionattorneys.org

Association of Administrators of the
Interstate Compact on
Adoption and Medical Assistance
810 First Street, N.E.
Suite 500
Washington, DC 20002
202-682-0100
http://aaicama.aphsa.org

FACE (Families Adopting
Children Everywhere)
Face, Inc.
P.O. Box 28058
Baltimore, MD 21239
410-488-2656 (Help-line)
www.faceadoptioninfo.org

Families for Private Adoption
P.O. Box 6375
Washington DC 20015-0375
202-722-0338
www.ffpa.org

Family Pride Coalition
P.O. Box 65327
Washington, DC 20035
202-231-5015
www.familypride.org

Generations United
1333 H Street, N.W.
Suite 500 W
Washington, DC 20005
202-289-3979
www.gu.org

Grandparents as Parents
P.O. 964
Lakewood, CA 90714
310-924-3996

International Concerns Committee for Children
911 Cypress Drive
Boulder, CO 80303
303-494-8333
www.iccadopt.org

Joint Council on International Children's Services
1403 King Street
Suite 101
Alexandria, VA 22314
703-535-8045
www.jcics.org

National Adoption Assistance Training Resource and Information Network
970 Raymond Avenue
Suite 106
St. Paul, MN 55114
800-470-6665

National Adoption Foundation
100 Mill Plain Road
Danbury, CT 06811
www.nafadopt.org/default.asp

National Adoption Information Clearinghouse
330 C Street, S.W.
Washington, DC 20447
888-251-0075
703-352-3488
www.calib.com/home

National Council for Adoption
225 North Washington Street
Alexandria, VA 22314
703-299-6633
www.adoptioncouncil.org

National Council for Single Adoptive Parents
P.O. Box 55
Wharton, NJ 07885
www.adopting.org/ncsap.html

National Resource Center for Special Needs Adoption
16250 Northland Drive
Suite 120
Southfield, MI 48075
248-443-0306
www.nrcadoption.org/index.htm

*North American Council on
Adoptable Children*
970 Raymond Avenue
Suite 106
St. Paul, MN 55114-1149
651-644-3036

Websites

Infertility

American Association of Tissue Banks
www.aath.org

*American Society of Reproductive
Medicine*
www.asrm.org

The American Surrogacy Center
(surrogacy and egg donor
information)
www.surrogacy.com

*Child of My Dreams:
Adoption and Infertility Support*
www.childofmydreams.com

*Children of Lesbians and
Gays Everywhere*
www.colage.org

Egg Donor Agencies
www.everythingsurrogacy.com

Embryo Adoption
www.fertilityplus.org/faq/
donor.html#embryo

Everything Surrogacy
www.everythingsurrogacy.com

Flexible Spending Account Calculator
www.principal.com/grouplh/
selffunded/fsacalculator.htm

*Flexible Spending Account
Regulations*
www.irs.gov/publications/p502/
index.html

Growing Generations (gay surrogacy)
www.growinggenerations.com

Home Insemination
www.fertilityplus.org

Human Clone Rights Foundation
www.humanclonerights.org
(coming soon)

IVF Connections Support
www.ivfconnections.com

Intended Parents
www.intendedparents.com

In Vitro Maturation
www.fertilitytutorials.com/
procedures_members/in_vitro_
matur_eggs.cfm

National Embryo Donation Center
www.embryodonation.org

*Offspring: for children seeking
sperm donor parents*
www.cbc.ca/programs/sites/
features/offspring/index.htm

Online Infertility Support Groups
www.surrogacy.com

Reprotech
(embryo donation info)
www.reprot.com

Single Mothers By Choice
http://mattes.home.pipeline.com

Sperm Bank Directory
www.spermbankdirectory.com

Sperm Bank List
www.fertilityplus.org/faq/
donor.html#sperm

Surrogate Mothers Online
www.surromomsonline.com

Adoption

Adoption Groups
www.adoptiongroups.com

Adoption Laws
www.law.cornell.edu/topics/
adoption.html

Adoption Online Support Group
www.adoptioncommunity.com

Adoption Support Group Database
www.adoptivefamilies.com/
support_group.php

*American Association of
Open Adoption Agencies*
www.openadoption.org

Association of Multiethnic Americans
www.ameasite.org

Child of My Dreams: Adoption and
Infertility Support
www.childofmydreams.com

Children of Lesbians and
Gays Everywhere
www.colage.org

Child Welfare League of America
www.cwla.org

Choosing an Adoption Agency
www.adoptivefamilies.com/
articles.php?aid=308

Comeunity Adoption Support
www.comeunity.com

Developmental Evaluators for
International Adoptions
www.adoption-research.org/
favorite.html

Domestic versus International
Adoption
www.adoptall.com/intguide.html

Families With Children From China
www.fwcc.org/welcome.html

Families with Children from Vietnam
www.fcvn.org

Foster Care Adoption
www.DaveThomasFoundationfor
Adoption.org

Gay and Lesbian-Friendly
Adoption Agencies
www.hrc.org

Home Study Agencies by State
www.siblingsadoption.com/
homestudyagency.htm

How to Make Adoption Affordable
www.nefe.org/adoption/index.ht
ml

International Adoptions
Finalized Abroad
www.calib.com/home

Joint Council of International
Children's Services
www.jcics.org

La leche League
www.laleche.org

Medicaid
www.cms.hhs.gov/medicaid

*National Adoption
Information Clearinghouse*
(division of the U.S. Department
of Health and Human Services)
www.calib.com/home

*National Dissemination Center
for Children w/ Disabilities*
www.nichcy.org

Older Child Adoption
www.olderchildadoption.com

Open Adoption Resources
www.r2press.com

Single Parent Adoption Network
http://members.aol.com/
Onemomfor2

*State Child Welfare Agencies and
Photolisting Sites*
www.calib.com/home

US Adoption laws by State
www.abcadoptions.com/uslaw.htm

US Department of State
www.state.gov

US Photolistings
www.adoptuskids.org/servlet/
page?_pageid=65&_dad=
portal30&_schema=PORTAL30

Appendix B

Forms

The following forms will be useful for different adoption and fertility arrangements. You can also find the adoption forms online at **http://uscis.gov**.

Insemination Agreement

This agreement is made on _____ (date) between the parties _____ (the donor) and _____ (the recipient).

1. The parties are both single and never married.

2. The donor agrees to provide semen to the recipient for use in artificial insemination.

3. The parties agree that the semen may be frozen and saved for future use and may also be used immediately.

4. The recipient agrees to pay the donor $_____ for each semen donation he makes under the terms of this agreement.

5. The parties agree that the donor is making donations for use by the recipient in her attempts to become pregnant. The recipient plans to use artificial insemination of the donor's semen during the following time period _____ to become pregnant.

6. The donor is donating semen for the recipient's use and agrees not to seek custody, visitation, guardianship, or contact with any child that results from the insemination. He hereby waives any and all parental rights now or in the future and waives any right as to the names of the children resulting from the insemination.

7. The donor agrees that she has no right to seek financial assistance from the donor and waives all rights to child support, confinement expenses or birth expenses for herself or any resulting child.

8. Both parties agree not to seek a determination of paternity of any child resulting from the insemination in any court or tribunal and waive any right to any such determination of paternity.

9. The parties agree that the birth certificates for any children resulting from the insemination will not name a father and specifically will not name the donor in any capacity.

10. The parties agree to use a licensed physician to perform the insemination. This is in compliance with _____ (fill in state law if applicable) to avoid the donor being named as the legal father of the child.

initial: _____   _____

11. The identity of the donor will be kept secret by both the donor and recipient and will not be revealed with consent of the other party.

12. The recipient shall have the right to choose a guardian for any children resulting from the insemination. The recipient shall also have the right to consent to a second-parent adoption of any children resulting from the insemination. Donor shall in no way interfere with any of these procedures, determinations, or exercises of rights.

13. The parties agree that the termination of rights stated in this agreement are permanent and irrevocable. Neither party may institute any court proceeding involving custody, visitation, guardianship, paternity, or child support against the other with respect to the children resulting from the insemination.

14. Donor agrees not to have any contact with any children resulting from the insemination without the express knowing consent of the recipient. The parties agree that any contact between donor and the resulting children shall in no way alter, impact, or effect the terms of this agreement or the legal relationship of the parties. Any contact that may occur will in no way be seen as implying or allowing donor the right to obtain, seek, or ask for parental rights or responsibilities.

15. The parties make this agreement willingly and freely, under no duress. Both parties have been advised to seek separate legal counsel before executing this document.

16. The parties understand each and every provision of this agreement. The agreement contains the entire agreement made between the parties and there are no other promises, understandings, or agreements between the parties other than what is contained herein.

17. The numbered provisions of this agreement may be enforced separately and individually by both parties.

18. This agreement is made pursuant to the laws of _____ [your state] and will be enforced according to the laws of that state.

initial: _____   _____

19. The parties agree that this agreement can only be altered in writing and must be signed by both parties to become valid.

_____   _____   _____

Donor Name   Donor Signature   Date

_____   _____   _____

Recipient Name   Recipient Signature   Date

Notary:

OMB NO. 1115-0049

U.S. Department of Justice
Immigration and Naturalization Service

Petition to Classify Orphan as an Immediate Relative

1. Eligibility.

A. Child. Under immigration law, an orphan is an alien child who has no parents because of the death or disappearance of, abandonment or desertion by, or separation or loss from both parents. An orphan is also a child who has only one parent who is not capable of taking care of the orphan and who has, in writing, irrevocably released the orphan for emigration and adoption. A petition to classify an alien as an orphan may not be filed in behalf of a child in the United States, unless that child is in parole status and has not been adopted in the United States. The petition must be filed before the child's 16th birthday.

B. Parent(s). The petition may be filed by a married United States citizen and spouse or unmarried United States citizen at least twenty-five years of age. The spouse does not need to be a United States citizen.

C. Adoption abroad. If the orphan was adopted abroad, it must be established that both the married petitioner and spouse or the unmarried petitioner personally saw and observed the child prior to or during the adoption proceedings. The adoption decree must show that a married petitioner and spouse adopted the child jointly or that an unmarried petitioner was at least 25 years of age at the time of the adoption.

D. Proxy adoption abroad. If both the petitioner and spouse or the unmarried petitioner did not personally see and observe the child prior to or during the adoption proceedings abroad, the petitioner (and spouse, if married) must submit a statement indicating the petitioner's (and, if married, the spouse's) willingness and intent to readopt the child in the United States. If requested, the petitioner must submit a statement by an official of the state in which the child will reside that readoption is permissible in that state. In addition, evidence of compliance with the preadoption requirements, if any, of that state must be submitted.

E. Preadoption requirements. If the orphan has not been adopted abroad, the petitioner and spouse or the unmarried petitioner must establish that the child will be adopted in the United States by the petitioner and spouse jointly or by the unmarried petitioner and that the preadoption requirement, if any, of the state of the orphan's proposed residence have been met.

2. Filing petition for known child.

An orphan petition for a child who has been identified must be submitted on a completed Form I-600 with the certification of petitioner executed and the required fee. If the petitioner is married, the Form I-600 must also be signed by the petitioner's spouse. The petition must be accompanied by the following:

A. Proof of United States citizenship of the petitioner.

(1) If the petitioner is a citizen by reason of birth in the United States, submit a copy of the petitioner's birth certificate, or if birth certificate is unobtainable, a copy of petitioner's baptismal certificate under the seal of the church, showing place of birth, (baptism must have occurred within two months after birth), or if a birth or baptismal certificate cannot be obtained, affidavits of two United States citizens who have personal knowledge of petitioner's birth in the United States.

(2) If the petitioner was born outside the United States and became a citizen through the naturalization or citizenship of a parent or husband and and has not been issued a certificate of citizenship in his or her own name, submit evidence of the citizenship and marriage of the parent or husband, as well as termination of any prior marriages.

Also, if petitioner claims citizenship through a parent, submit petitioner's birth certificate and a separate statement showing the date, place, and means of all his or her arrivals and departures into and out of the United States.

(3) If petitioner's naturalization occurred within 90 days immediately preceding the filing of this petition, or if it occurred prior to September 27, 1906, the naturalization certificate must accompany the petition.

(4) An unexpired, U.S. passport initially issued for ten years may also be submitted.

B. Proof of marriage of petitioner and spouse.
The married petitioner should submit a certificate of the marriage and proof of termination of all prior marriages of himself or herself and spouse. In the case of an unmarried petitioner who was previously married, submit proof of termination of all prior marriages. **NOTE:** If any change occurs in the petitioner's marital status while the case is pending, the district director should be notified immediately.

C. Proof of age of orphan.
Petitioner should submit a copy of the orphan's birth certificate if obtainable; if not obtainable, submit an explanation together with the best available evidence of birth.

D. Copies of the death certificate(s) of the child's parent(s), if applicable.

E. A certified copy of adoption decree together with certified translation, if the orphan has been lawfully adopted abroad.

F. Evidence that the sole or surviving parent is incapable of providing for the orphan's care and has, in writing, irrevocably released the orphan for emigration and adoption, if the orphan has only one parent.

G. Evidence that the orphan has been unconditionally abandoned to an orphanage, if the orphan has been placed in an orphanage by his/her parent or parents.

H. Evidence that the preadoption requirements, if any, of the state of the orphan's proposed residence have been met, if the child is to be adopted in the United States. If it is not possible to submit this evidence upon initial filing of the petition under the laws of the state of proposed residence, it may be submitted later. The petition, however, will not be approved without it.

I. A home study with a statement or attachment recommending or approving of the adoption or proposed adoption signed by an official of the responsible state agency in the state of the child's proposed residence or of an agency authorized by that state, or, in the case of a child adopted abroad, of an appropriate public or private adoption agency which is licensed in the United States. Both individuals and organizations may qualify as agencies. If the recommending agency is a licensed agency, the recommendation must set forth that it is licensed, the state in which it is licensed, its license number, if any, and the period of validity of its license. The research, including interviewing, however, and the preparation of the home study may be done by an individual or group in the United States or abroad satisfactory to the recommending agency. A responsible state agency or licensed agency can accept a home study made by an unlicensed agency can accept a home study made by an unlicensed or foreign agency and use that home study as a basis for a favorable recommendation. The home study must contain, but is not limited to, the following elements:

(1) the financial ability of the adoptive or prospective parent or parents to read and educate the child.

(2) a detailed description of the living accommodations where the adoptive or prospective parent or parents currently reside.

(3) a detailed description of the living accommodations where the child will reside.

(4) a factual evaluation of the physical, mental, and moral capabilities of the adoptive or prospective parent or parents in relation to rearing and educating the child.

J. **Fingerprints.**
Each member of the married prospective adoptive couple or the married prospective adoptive parent, and each additional adult member of the prospective adoptive parents' household must be fingerprinted in connection with this petition.

Petitioners residing in the United States. After filing this petition, INS will notify each person in writing of the time and location where they must go to be fingerprinted. Failure to appear to be fingerprinted may result in denial of the petition.

Petitioners residing abroad. Completed fingerprint cards (Forms FD-258) must be submitted with the petition. Do not bend, fold, or crease completed fingerprint cards. Fingerprint cards must be prepared by a United States consular office or a United States military installation.

3. **Filing Petition for Known Child Without Full Documentation on Child or Home Study.**
When a child has been identified but the documentary evidence relating to him/her or the home study is not yet available, an orphan petition may be filed without that evidence or home study. The evidence outlined in Instructions 2A and 2B, however, must be submitted. If the necessary evidence relating to the child or the home study is not submitted within one year from the date of submission of the petition, the petition will be considered abandoned and the fee will not be refunded. Any further proceeding will require the filing of a new petition.

4. **Submitting an Application for Advance Processing of an Orphan Petition in Behalf of a Child Who Has Not Been Identified.**
A prospective petitioner may request advance processing when the child has not been identified or when the prospective petitioner and/or spouse are or is going abroad to locate or adopt a child. If unmarried, the prospective petitioner must be at least 24 years of age, provided that he or she will be at least 25 at the time of the adoption and the completed petition in behalf of a child is filed. The request must be on Form I-600A, Application for Advance Processing of Orphan Petition, and must be accompanied by the evidence required by that form. After a child or children are located and/or identified, a separate Form I-600, Petition to Classify Orphan as an Immediate Relative, must be filed for each child. A new fee is not required if only one Form I-600 is filed, provided the form is filed within one year of completion of all advance

processing in a case where there has been a favorable determination concerning the prospective petitioner's ability to care for a beneficiary orphan.

5. **When Child/Children Located and/or Identified.**
A separate form I-600, Petition to Classify Orphan as an Immediate Relative, must be filed for each child. A new fee is not required if only one form I-600 is filed and it is filed within one year of completion of all advance processing in a case where there has been a favorable determination concerning the beneficiary orphan.

Normally, Form I-600 should be submitted to the INS office where the advance processing application was filed. The Immigration and Naturalization Service has offices in the following countries: Austria, China, Cuba, Denmark, Dominican Republic, Ecuador, El Salvador, Germany, Ghana, Great Britain, Greece, Guatemala, Haiti, Honduras, India, Italy, Jamaica, Kenya, Korea, Mexico, Pakistan, Panama, Peru, Philippines, Russia, Singapore, South Africa, Spain, Thailand, and Vietnam. A prosepective petitioner who is going abroad to adopt or locate a child in one of these countries should file Form I-600 at the INS office having jurisdiction over the place where the child is residing or will be located unless the case is being retained at the stateside office.

However, a prospective petitioner who is going abroad to any other country to adopt or locate a child should file Form I-600 at the American embassy or consulate having jurisdiction over the place where the child is residing or wil be located unless the case is being retained at the stateside office.

The case may be retained at the stateside office, if the petitioner requests it and if it appears that the case will be processed more quickly in that manner. Form I-600 must be accompanied by all the evidence required on the instruction sheet of that form, except that the evidence required by and submitted with this form need not be furnished.

6. **General Filing Instructions.**
A. Type or print legibly in ink.

B. If extra space is needed to complete any item, attach a continuation sheet, indicate the item number, and date and sign each sheet.

C. **Translations.** Any foreign language document must be accompanied by a full English translation, which the translator has certified as complete and correct, and by the translator's certification that he or she is competent to translate the foreign language into English.

D. **Copies.** If these instruction state that a copy of a document may be filed with this petition and you choose to send us the original, we may keep that original for our records.

7. Submission of petition.

A petitioner residing in the United States should send the completed petition to the INS office having jurisdiction over his/her place of residence. A petitioner residing outside the United States should consult the nearest American embassy or consulate designated to act on the petition.

8. Fee. Read instructions carefully.

A fee of four hundred and sixty dollars ($460) must be submitted for filing this petition. There is a fifty dollar ($50) per person, fingerprinting fee, in addition to the petition fee for each person residing in the United States and required to be fingerprinted. For example, if a petition is filed by a married couple residing in the United States with one additional adult member in their household, the total of fees that must be submitted is $610. However, if a petition is filed by a married couple residing abroad, only the petition fee of $460 must be submitted.

One check or money order may be submitted for both the petition fee and the fingerprinting fees. It cannot be refunded regardless of the action taken on the petition. **Do not mail cash. All fees must be submitted in the exact amount.** Payment by a check or money order must be drawn on a bank or other institution located in the United States and be payable in United States currency.

If the petitioner resides in Guam, the check or money order must be payable to the "Treasurer, Guam."

If the petitioner resides in the Virgin Islands, check or money order must be payable to the "Commissioner of Finance of the Virgin Islands."

All other petitioners must make the check or money order payable to the "Immigration and Naturalization Service." When a check is drawn on the account of a person other than the petitioner, the name of the petitioner must be entered on the face of the check.

If petition is submitted from outside the United States, remittance may be made by a bank international money order or foreign draft drawn on a financial institution in the United States and payable to the Immigration and Naturalization Service in United States currency. Personal checks are accepted subject to collectibility. An uncollectible check in payment of a petition fee will render the petition and any document issued invalid. A charge of $30.00 will be imposed if a check in payment of a fee is not honored by the bank on which it is drawn. When more than one petition is submitted by the same petitioner in behalf of orphans who are siblings, only one set of petition and fingerprinting fees is required.

9. Assistance.

Assistance may be obtained from a recognized social agency or from any public or private agency. The following recognized social agencies, which have offices in many of the principal cities of the United States, have agreed to furnish assistance:

Bethany Christian Services.
2600 Fivemile Road NE
Grand Rapids, MI. 419525
Tel: (616) 224-7446
Fax: (616) 224-7585

Catholic Legal Immigration Network, Inc., (CLINIC).
415 Michigan Avenue, NE., Suite 150
Washington, DC 20017
Tel: (202) 635-2556
Fax: (202) 635-2649

International Social Services/U.S. of America Branch
700 Light Street
Baltimore, MD. 21230
Tel: (410) 230-2734
Fax: (410) 230-2741

United States Catholic Conference Migration and Refugee Services (USCC/MRS).
3211 4th Street, NE
Washington, DC 20017
Tel: (202) 541-3352
Fax: (202) 722-8800

10. Penalties.

Willful false statements on this form or supporting documents can be punished by fine or imprisonment. U.S. Code, Title 18, Sec. 1001 (formerly Sec. 80.)

11 Authority.

8 USC 1154(a). Routine uses for disclosure under the Privacy Act of 1974 have been published in the Federal Register and are available upon request. INS will use the information to determine immigrant eligibility. Submission of the information is voluntary, but failure to provide any or all of the information may result in denial of the petition.

12 Reporting Burden.

A person is not required to respond to a collection of information unless it displays a currently valid OMB control number. Public reporting burden for this collection of information is estimated to average 30 minutes per response, including the time for reviewing instructions, searching existing data sources, gathering and maintaining the data needed, and completing and reviewing the collection of information. Send comments regarding this burden estimate or any other aspect of this collection of information, including suggestions for reducing this burden, to: Immigration and Naturalization Service, HQPDI, 425 I Street, N.W., Room 4034, Washington, DC 20536; OMB No. 1115-0049. **DO NOT MAIL YOUR COMPLETED APPLICATION TO THIS ADDRESS.**

OMB No. 1115-0049

Petition to Classify Orphan as
an Immediate Relative

U.S. Department of Justice
Immigration and Naturalization Service

[Section 101 (b)(1)(F) of the Immigration and Nationality Act, as amended.]

Please do not write in this block.

TO THE SECRETARY OF STATE;
The petition was filed by:

☐ Married petitioner   ☐ Unmarried petitioner

The petition is approved for orphan:

☐ Adopted abroad   ☐ Coming to U.S. for adoption.
Preadoption requirements have
been met.

Remarks:

Fee Stamp

File number

DATE OF
ACTION

DD

DISTRICT

Please type or print legibly in ink. Use a separate petition for each child.

Petition is being made to classify the named orphan as an immediate relative.

BLOCK I - Information about prospective

1. My name is: (Last)   (First)   (Middle)

2. Other names used (including maiden name if appropriate):

3. I reside in the U.S.   (C/O if appropriate)   (Apt. No.)

   (Number and street)   (Town or city)   (State)   (Zip Code)

4. Address abroad (if any)(Number and street)   (Apt. No.)

   (Town or city)   (Province)   (Country)

5. I was born on: (Month)   (Day)   (Year)

   In: (Town or City)   (State or Province)   (Country)

6. My phone number is: (Include Area Code)

7. My marital status is:
   ☐ Married
   ☐ Widowed
   ☐ Divorced
   ☐ Single
      ☐ I have never been married.
      ☐ I have been previously married _____ time(s).

8. If you are now married, give the following information:

   Date and place of present marriage

   Name of present spouse (include maiden name of wife)

   Date of birth of spouse   Place of birth of spouse

   Number of prior marriages of spouse

   My spouse resides ☐ With me   ☐ Apart from me
   (provide address below)
   (Apt. No.)   (No. and street)   (City)   (State)   (Country)

9. I am a citizen of the United States through:
   ☐ Birth   ☐ Parents   ☐ Naturalization
   If acquired through naturalization, give name under which
   naturalized, number of naturalization certificate, and date and
   place of naturalization:

   If not, submit evidence of citizenship. See Instruction 2.a(2).
   If acquired through parentage, have you obtained a certificate in
   your own name based on that acquisition?
   ☐ No   ☐ Yes

   Have you or any person through whom you claimed citizenship
   ever lost United States citizenship?
   ☐ No   ☐ Yes (If yes, attach detailed explanation.)

Continue on reverse.

Received	Trans. In	Ret'd Trans. Out	Completed

Form I-600 (Rev. 11/28/01)Y Page 1

BLOCK II - Information about orphan beneficiary

10. Name at birth   (First)   (Middle)   (Last)

11. Name at present   (First)   (Middle)   (Last)

12. Any other names by which orphan is or was known.

13. Sex   ☐ Male
           ☐ Female

14. Date of birth (Month/Day/Year)

15. Place of birth (City)   (State or Province)   (Country)

16. The beneficiary is an orphan because (check One)
    ☐ He/she has no parents.
    ☐ He/she has only one parent who is the sole or surviving

17. If the orphan has only one parent, answer the following
    a. State what has become of the other parent:

    b. Is the remaining parent capable of providing for the orphan's
       support?   ☐ Yes   ☐ No
    c. Has the remaining parent, in writing, irrevocably released
       orphan for emigration and adoption? ☐ Yes   ☐ No

18. Has the orphan been adopted abroad by the petitioner and
    jointly or the unmarried petitioner?   ☐ Yes   ☐ No

    If yes, did the petitioner and spouse or unmarried petitioner
    personally see and observe the child prior to or during the
    adoption proceedings?   ☐ Yes   ☐ No

    Date of adoption

    Place of adoption

19. If either answer in question 18 is "No", answer the following:
    a. Do petitioner and spouse jointly or does the unmarried
        intend to adopt the orphan in the United States?
                              ☐ Yes   ☐ No
    b. Have the preadoption requirements, if any, of the orphan's
        proposed state of residence been met?
                              ☐ Yes   ☐ No
    c. If b. is answered "No", will they be met later?
                              ☐ Yes   ☐ No

20. To petitioner's knowledge, does the orphan have any physical or
    affliction?   ☐ Yes   ☐ No

    If "Yes", name the affliction.

21. Who has legal custody of the child?

22. Name of child welfare agency, if any, assisting in this case:

23. Name of attorney abroad, if any, representing petitioner in this

    Address of above.

24. Address in the United States where orphan will reside.

25. Present address of orphan.

25. If orphan is residing in an institution, give full name of institution.

26. If orphan is not residing in an institution, give full name of person
    whom orphan is residing.

27. Give any additional information necessary to locate orphan such
    as name of district, section, zone or locality in which orphan
    resides.

28. Location of American Consulate where application for visa will
    be made.
    (City in Foreign Country)   (Foreign Country)

Certification of prospective petitioner
I certify under penalty of perjury under the laws of the United
States of America that the foregoing is true and correct and that
I will care for an orphan/orphans properly if admitted to the
United States.

(Signature of Prospective Petitioner)

Executed on (Date)

Certification of married prospective petitioner's spouse
I certify under penalty of perjury under the laws of the United
States of America that the foregoing is true and correct and that
my spouse and I will care for an orphan/orphans properly if
admitted to the United States.

(Signature of Prospective Petitioner)

Executed on (Date)

Signature of person preparing form, if other than petitioner
I declare that this document was prepared by me at the request of the
prospective petitioner and is based on all information of which I have
any knowledge.

(Signature)

Address

Executed on (Date)

OMB No. 1115-0049

U.S. Department of Justice
Immigration and Naturalization Service

Application for Advance Processing of Orphan Petition (8CFR 204.1(b)(3))

Advanced processing is a procedure for completing the part of an orphan petition relating to the petitioner before an orphan is located so that there will be no unnecessary delays in processing the petition after an orphan is located. **USE THIS FORM ONLY IF YOU WISH TO ADOPT AN ORPHAN WHO HAS NOT YET BEEN LOCATED AND IDENTIFIED OR YOU AND/OR YOUR SPOUSE, IF MARRIED, ARE/IS GOING ABROAD TO ADOPT OR LOCATE A CHILD.** This application is not a petition to classify orphan as an immediate relative (Form I-600).

1. Eligibility.

A. Eligibility for advance processing application (Form I-600A). An application for advance processing may be filed by a married United States citizen and spouse. The spouse does not need to be a United States citizen. It may also be filed by an unmarried United States citizen at least 24 years of age provided that he or she will be at least 25 at the time of the adoption and of filing an orphan petition in behalf of a child.

B. Eligibility for Orphan Petition (Form I-600). In addition to the requirements concerning the citizenship and age of the petitioner described in Instruction 1a, when a child is located and identified, the following eligibility requirements will apply:

(1) **Child.** Under immigration law, an orphan is an alien child who has no parents because of the death or disappearance of, abandonment or desertion by, or separation or loss from both parents. An orphan is also a child who has only one parent who is not capable of taking care of the orphan and who has, in writing, irrevocably released the orphan for emigration and adoption. A petition to classify an alien as an orphan may not be filed in behalf of a child in the United States unless that child is in parole status and has not been adopted in the United States. The petition must be filed before the child's 16th birthday.

(2) **Adoption abroad.** If the orphan was adopted abroad, it must be established that both the married petitioner and spouse or the unmarried petitioner personally saw and observed the child prior to or during the adoption proceedings. The adoption decree must show that a married petitioner and spouse adopted the child jointly or that an unmarried petitioner was at least 25 years of age at the time of the adoption.

(3) **Proxy adoption abroad.** If both the petitioner and spouse or the unmarried petitioner did not personally see and observe the child prior to or during the adoption proceedings abroad, the petitioner (and spouse, if married) must submit a statement indicating the petitioner's (and, if married, the spouse's) willingness and intent to readopt the child in the United States. If requested, the petitioner must submit a statement by an official of the state in which the child will reside that readoption is permissible in that state. In addition, evidence of compliance with the preadoption requirements, if any, of that state must be submitted.

(4) **Preadoption requirements.** If the orphan has not been adopted abroad, the petitioner and spouse or the unmarried petitioner must establish that the child will be adopted in the United States by the petitioner and spouse jointly or by the unmarried petitioner and that the preadoption requirement, if any, of the state of the orphan's proposed residence have been met.

2. Filing Advance Processing Application.

An advance processing application must be submitted on Form I-600A with the certification of prospective petitioner executed and the required fee. If the prospective petitioner is married, the Form I-600A must also be signed by the prospective petitioner's spouse. The application must be accompanied by:

A. Proof of United States citizenship of the prospective petitioner.

(1) If the petitioner is a citizen by reason of birth in the United States, submit a copy of the petitioner's birth certificate, or if birth certificate is unobtainable, a copy of petitioner's baptismal certificate under seal of the church, showing place of birth, (baptism must have occurred within two months after birth), or if a birth or baptismal certificate cannot be obtained, affidavits of two United States citizens who have personal knowledge of petitioner's birth in the United States.

(2) If the petitioner was born outside the United States and became a citizen through the naturalization or citizenship of a parent or husband and has not been issued a certificate of citizenship in his or her own name, submit evidence of the citizenship and marriage of the parent or husband, as well as termination of any prior marriages. Also, if petitioner claims citizenship through a parent, submit a copy of the petitioner's birth certificate and a separate statement showing the date, place, and means of all his/her arrivals and departures into and out of the United States.

(3) If petitioner's naturalization occurred within 90 days immediately preceding the filing of this petition, or if it occurred prior to September 27, 1906, a copy of the naturalization certificate must accompany the petition.

(4) An unexpired U.S. passport initially issued for ten years may also be submitted.

B. Proof of marriage of petitioner and spouse.
The married petitioner should submit a copy of the certificate of the marriage and proof of termination of all prior marriages of himself or herself and spouse. In the case of an unmarried petitioner who was previously married, submit proof of termination of all prior marriages. **NOTE:** If any change occurs in the petitioner's marital status while the case is pending, the district director should be notified immediately.

C. A **home study** with a statement or attachment recommending or approving of the adoption or proposed adoption signed by an official of the responsible state agency in the state of the child's proposed residence or of an agency authorized by that state, or, in the case of a child adopted abroad, of an appropriate public or private adoption agency which is licensed in the United States. Both individuals and organizations may qualify as agencies. If the recommending agency is a licensed agency, the recommendation must set forth that it is licensed, the state in which it is licensed, its license number, if any, and the period of validity of its license. The research, including interviewing, however, and the preparation of the home study may be done by an individual or group in the United States or abroad satisfactory to the recommending agency. A responsible state agency or licensed agency can accept a home study made by an unlicensed or foreign agency and use that home study as a basis for a favorable recommendation. The home study must contain, but is not limited to, the following elements:

(1) the financial ability of the adoptive or prospective parent or parents to rear and educate the child.

(2) a detailed description of the living accommodations where the adoptive or prospective parent or parents currently reside.

(3) A detailed description of the living accommodations where the child will reside.

(4) A factual evaluation of the physical, mental, and moral capabilities of the adoptive or prospective parent or parents in relation to rearing and educating the child.

D. Fingerprints.
Each member of the married prospective adoptive couple or the married prospective adoptive parent, and each additional adult member of the prospective adoptive parents' household must be fingerprinted in connection with this petition.

(1) *Petitioners residing in the United States.* After filing this petition, INS will notify each person in writing of the time and location where they must go to be fingerprinted. Failure to appear to be fingerprinted may result in denial of the petition.

(2) *Petitioners residing Abroad.* Completed fingerprint cards (Forms FD-258)

must be submitted with the petition. Do not bend, fold, or crease completed fingerprint cards. Fingerprint cards must be prepared by a United States consular office or a United States military installation.

3. General Filing Instructions.

A. Type or print legibly in ink.

B. If extra space is needed to complete any item, attach a continuation sheet, indicate the item number, and date and sign each sheet.

C. Translations. Any foreign language document must be accompanied by a full English translation, which the translator has certified as complete and correct, and by the translator's certification that he or she is competent to translate the foreign language into English.

D. Copies. If these instructions state that a copy of a document may be filed with this petition and you choose to send us the original, we may keep that original for our records.

4. Submission of Application.

A prospective petitioner residing in the United States should send the completed application to the office of this Service having jurisdiction over his or her place of residence. A prospective petitioner residing outside the United States should consult the nearest American consulate for the overseas or stateside INS office designated to act on the application.

5. Fee. (Read instructions carefully.)

A fee of four hundred and sixty dollars ($460) must be submitted for filing this petition. There is a fifty dollar ($50) per person fingerprinting fee in addition to the petition fee for each person residing in the United States and required to be fingerprinted. For example, if a petition is filed by a married couple residing in the United States with one additional adult member in their household, the total of fees that must be submitted is $610. However, if a petition is filed by a married couple residing abroad, only the petition fee of $460 must be submitted.

One check or money order may be submitted for both the petition fee and the fingerprinting fees. All fees must be submitted in the exact amount. Payment by check or money order must be drawn on a bank or other institution located in the

United States and be payable in United States currency.

If petitioner resides in Guam, the check or money order must be payable to the "Treasurer, Guam."

If petitioner resides in the Virgin Islands, the check or money order must be payable to the "Commissioner of Finance of the Virgin Islands."

All other petitioners must make the check or money order payable to the "Immigration and Naturalization Service." When a check is drawn on the account of a person other than the petitioner, the name of the petitioner must be entered on the face of the check.

If petition is submitted from outside the United States, remittance may be made by bank international money order or foreign draft drawn on a financial institution in the United States and payable to the Immigration and Naturalization Service in United States currency. Personal checks are accepted subject to collectibility. An uncollectible check in payment of a petition fee will render the petition and any document issued invalid. A charge of $30.00 will be imposed if a check in payment of a fee is not honored by the bank on which it is drawn.

When more than one petition is submitted by the same petitioner in behalf of orphans who are siblings, only one set of petition and fingerprinting fees is required.

6. When Child/Children Located and/or Identified.

A separate Form I-600, Petition to Classify Orphan as an Immediate Relative, must be filed for each child. A new fee is not required if only one form I-600 is filed and it is filed within one year of completion of all advance processing in a case where there has been a favorable determination concerning the beneficiary orphan.

Normally, Form I-600 should be submitted to the INS office where the advance processing application was filed. The immigration and Naturalization Service has offices in the following countries: Austria, China, Cuba, Denmark, Domincan Republic, Ecuador, El Salvador, Germany, Ghana, Great Britain, Greece, Guatemala, Haiti, Honduras, India, Italy, Jamaica, Kenya, Korea, Mexico, Pakistan, Panama, Peru, Philippines, Russia, Singapore, South Africa, Spain, Thailand, and Vietnam. A prospective petitioner who is going abroad to adopt or locate a child in one of these countries should file Form I-600 at the INS office having jurisdiction over the place where the child is residing or will be located, unless the case is being retained at the stateside office.

However, a prospective petitioner who is going abroad to any other country to adopt or locate a child should file Form I-600 at the American consulate or embassy having jurisdiction over the place where the child is residing or will be located unless the case is being retained at the stateside office.

The case may be retained at the stateside office, if the petitioner requests it and if it appears that the case will be processed more quickly in that manner. Form I-600 must be accompanied by all the evidence required on the instruction sheet of that form, except that the evidence required by and submitted with this form need not be furnished.

Assistance.

Assistance may be obtained from a recognized social agency or from any public or private agency. The following recognized social agencies, which have offices in many of the principal cities of the United States, have agreed to furnish assistance:

Bethany Christian Services.
2600 Fivemile Road NE
Grand Rapids, MI. 49525
Tel: (616) 224-7446
Fax: (616) 224-7585

Catholic Legal Immigration Network, Inc. (CLINIC)
415 Michigan Avenue, NE., Suite 150
Washington, DC 20017
Tel: (202) 635-2556
Fax: (202) 632-2649

International Social Services/U.S. of America Branch.
700 Light Street
Baltimore, MD. 21230
Tel: (410) 230-2734
Fax: (410) 230-2741

United States Catholic Conference Migration and Refugee Services (USCC/MRS).
3211 4th Street, NE
Washington, DC 20017
Tel: (202) 541-3352
Fax: (202) 722-8800

8. Penalties.

Willful false statements on this form or supporting documents can be punished by fine or imprisonment. U.S. Code, Title 18, Sec. 1001 (Formerly Sec. 80.)

9. Authority.

8 U.S.C 1154(a). Routine uses for disclosure under the Privacy Act of 1974 have been published in the Federal Register and are available upon request. The Immigration and Naturalization Service will use the information to determine immigrant eligibility. Submission of the information is voluntary, but failure to provide any or all of the information may result in denial of the petition.

10. Reporting Burden.

A person is not required to respond to a collection of information unless it displays a currently valid OMB control number. Public reporting burden for this collection of information is estimated to average 30 minutes per response, including the time for reviewing instructions, searching existing data sources, gathering and maintaining the data needed, and completing and reviewing the collection of information. Send comments regarding this burden estimate or any other aspect of this collection of information, including suggestions for reducing this burden, to: Immigration and Naturalization Service, HQPDI, 425 I Street, N.W., Room 4034, Washington, DC 20536; OMB No. 1115-0049. **DO NOT MAIL YOUR COMPLETED APPLICATION TO THIS ADDRESS.**

OMB No. 1115-0049

U.S. Department of Justice
Immigration and Naturalization Service

Application for Advance Processing of Orphan Petition [8CFR 204.1(b)(3)]

Please do not write in this block.

It has been determined that the

☐ Married   ☐ Unmarried

Fee Stamp

There

☐ are   ☐ are not
preadoptive requirements in the state of the child's
proposed residence.

The following is a description of the preadoption requirements, if
any, of the state of the child's proposed residence:

DATE OF FAVORABLE
DETERMINATION

DD

DISTRICT

The preadoption requirements, if any,
☐ have been met.   ☐ have not been met.

File number of petitioner, if applicable

Please type or print legibly in ink.

Application is made by the named prospective petitioner for advance processing of an orphan petition.

BLOCK I - Information about prospective petitioner

1. My name is: (Last)   (First)   (Middle)

2. Other names used (including maiden name if appropriate):

3. I reside in the U.S. at: (C/O if appropriate)   (Apt. No.)

   (Number and street)   (Town or city)   (State)   (ZIP Code)

4. Address abroad (if any):   (Number and street)   (Apt. No.)

   (Town or city)   (Province)   (Country)

5. I was born on: (Month)   (Day)   (Year)

   In: (Town or City)   (State or Province)   (Country)

6. My phone number is: (Include Area Code)

7. My marital status is:
   ☐ Married
   ☐ Widowed
   ☐ Divorced
   ☐ Single
       ☐ I have never been married.
       ☐ I have been previously married _____ time(s).

8. If you are now married, give the following information:
   Date and place of present marriage

   Name of present spouse (include maiden name of wife)

   Date of birth of spouse   Place of birth of spouse

   Number of prior marriages of spouse

   My spouse resides ☐ With me   ☐ Apart from me
                                        (provide address below)
   (Apt. No.)   (No. and street)   (City)   (State)   (Country)

9. I am a citizen of the United States through:
       ☐ Birth   ☐ Parents   ☐ Naturalization
   If acquired through naturalization, give name under which
   naturalized, number of naturalization certificate, and date and
   place of naturalization.

   If not, submit evidence of citizenship. See Instruction 2.a(2).
   If acquired through parentage, have you obtained a certificate
   in your own name based on that acquisition?
       ☐ No   ☐ Yes
   Have you or any person through whom you claimed citizenship
   ever lost United States citizenship?
       ☐ No   ☐ Yes (If yes, attach detailed explanation.)

Continue on reverse.

Received	Trans. In	Ret'd Trans. Out	Completed

Form I-600A (Rev. 12/04/01)Y Page 1

BLOCK II - General information

10. Name and address of organization or individual assisting you in locating or identifying an orphan

(Name)

(Address)

11. Do you plan to travel abroad to locate or adopt a child?
☐ Yes ☐ No

12. Does your spouse, if any, plan to travel abroad to locate or adopt a child?
☐ Yes ☐ No

13. If the answer to question 11 or 12 is "yes," give the following information:

a. Your date of intended departure _____

b. Your spouse's date of intended departure _____

c. City, province _____

14. Will the child come to the United States for adoption after compliance with the preadoption requirements, if any, of the state of proposed residence?
☐ Yes ☐ No

15. If the answer to question 14 is "no," will the child be adopted abroad after having been personally seen and observed by you and your spouse, if married?
☐ Yes ☐ No

16. Where do you wish to file your orphan petition?

The service office located at

The American Embassy or Consulate at

17. Do you plan to adopt more than one child?
☐ Yes ☐ No

If "Yes", how many children do you plan to adopt?

Certification of prospective petitioner
I certify, under penalty of perjury under the laws of the United States of America, that the foregoing is true and correct and that I will care for an orphan/orphans properly if admitted to the United States.

(Signature of Prospective Petitioner)

Executed on (Date)

Certification of married prospective petitioner's spouse
I certify, under penalty of perjury under the laws of the United States of America, that the foregoing is true and correct and that my spouse and I will care for an orphan/orphans properly if admitted to the United States.

(Signature of Prospective Petitioner)

Executed on (Date)

Signature of person preparing form, if other than petitioner
I declare that this document was prepared by me at the request of the prospective petitioner and is based on all information of which I have any knowledge.

(Signature)

Address

Executed on (Date)

U.S. Department of Justice
Immigration and Naturalization Service

OMB No. 1115-0214

Affidavit of Support Under Section 213A of the Act

INSTRUCTIONS

Purpose of this Form

This form is required to show that an intending immigrant has adequate means of financial support and is not likely to become a public charge.

Sponsor's Obligation

The person completing this affidavit is the sponsor. A sponsor's obligation continues until the sponsored immigrant becomes a U.S. citizen, can be credited with 40 qualifying quarters of work, departs the United States permanently, or dies. Divorce does not terminate the obligation. By signing this form, you, the sponsor, agree to support the intending immigrant and any spouse and/or children immigrating with him or her and to reimburse any government agency or private entity that provides these sponsored immigrants with Federal, State, or local means-tested public benefits.

General Filing Instructions

Please answer all questions by typing or clearly printing in black ink only. Indicate that an item is not applicable with "N/A". If an answer is "none," please so state. If you need extra space to answer any item, attach a sheet of paper with your name and Social Security number, and indicate the number of the item to which the answer refers.

You must submit an affidavit of support for each applicant for immigrant status. You may submit photocopies of this affidavit for any spouse or children immigrating with an immigrant you are sponsoring. For purposes of this form, a spouse or child is immigrating with an immigrant you are sponsoring if he or she is: 1) listed in Part 3 of this affidavit of support; and 2) applies for an immigrant visa or adjustment of status within 6 months of the date this affidavit of support is originally completed and signed. The signature on the affidavit must be notarized by a notary public or signed before an Immigration or a Consular officer.

You should give the completed affidavit of support with all required documentation to the sponsored immigrant for submission to either a Consular Officer with Form OF-230, Application for Immigrant Visa and Alien Registration, or an Immigration Officer with Form I-485, Application to Register Permanent Residence or Adjust Status. You may enclose the affidavit of support and accompanying documents in a sealed envelope to be opened only by the designated Government official. The sponsored immigrant must submit the affidavit of support to the Government within 6 months of its signature.

Who Needs an Affidavit of Support under Section 213A?

This affidavit must be filed at the time an intending immigrant is applying for an immigrant visa or adjustment of status. It is required for:

- All immediate relatives, including orphans, and family-based immigrants. (Self-petitioning widow/ers and battered spouses and children are exempt from this requirement); and

- Employment-based immigrants where a relative filed the immigrant visa petition or has a significant ownership interest (5 percent or more) in the entity that filed the petition.

Who Completes an Affidavit of Support under Section 213A?

- For immediate relatives and family-based immigrants, the family member petitioning for the intending immigrant must be the sponsor.

- For employment-based immigrants, the petitioning relative or a relative with a significant ownership interest (5 percent or more) in the petitioning entity must be the sponsor. The term "relative," for these purposes, is defined as husband, wife, father, mother, child, adult son or daughter, brother, or sister.

- If the petitioner cannot meet the income requirements, a joint sponsor may submit an additional affidavit of support.

A sponsor, or joint sponsor, must also be:

- A citizen or national of the United States or an alien lawfully admitted to the United States for permanent residence;

- At least 18 years of age; and

- Domiciled in the United States or its territories and possessions.

Sponsor's Income Requirement

As a sponsor, your household income must equal or exceed 125 percent of the Federal poverty line for your household size. For the purpose of the affidavit of support, household size includes yourself, all persons related to you by birth, marriage, or adoption living in your residence, your dependents, any immigrants you have previously sponsored using INS Form I-864 if that obligation has not terminated, and the intending immigrant(s) in Part 3 of this affidavit of support. The poverty guidelines are calculated and published annually by the Department of Health and Human Services. Sponsors who are on active duty in the U.S. Armed Forces other than for training need only demonstrate income at 100 percent of the poverty line *if* they are submitting this affidavit for the purpose of sponsoring their spouse or child.

If you are currently employed and have an *individual* income which meets or exceeds 125 percent of the Federal poverty line or (100 percent, if applicable) for your household size, you do not need to list the income of any other person. When determining your income, you may include the income generated by individuals related to you by birth, marriage, or adoption who are living in your residence, if they have lived in your residence for the previous 6 months, or who are listed as dependents on your most recent Federal income tax return whether or not they live in your residence. For their income to be considered, these household members or dependents must be willing to make their income available for the support of the sponsored immigrant(s) if necessary, and to complete and sign Form I-864A, Contract Between Sponsor and Household Member. However, a household member who is the immigrant you are sponsoring only need complete Form I-864A if his or her income will be used to determine your ability to support a spouse and/or children immigrating with him or her.

If in any of the most recent 3 tax years, you and your spouse each reported income on a joint income tax return, but you want to use only your own income to qualify (and your spouse is not submitting a Form I-864A), you may provide a separate breakout of your individual income for these years. Your individual income will be based on the earnings from your W-2 forms, Wage and Tax Statement, submitted to IRS for any such years. If necessary to meet the income requirement, you may also submit evidence of other income listed on your tax returns which can be attributed to you. You must provide documentation of such reported income, including Forms 1099 sent by the payer, which show your name and Social Security number.

You must calculate your household size and total household income as indicated in Parts 4.B. and 4.C. of this form. You must compare your total household income with the minimum income requirement for your household size using the poverty guidelines. For the purposes of the affidavit of support, determination of your ability to meet the income requirements will be based on the most recent poverty guidelines published in the Federal Register at the time the Consular or Immigration Officer makes a decision on the intending immigrant's application for an immigrant visa or adjustment of status. Immigration and Consular Officers will begin to use updated poverty guidelines on the first day of the second month after the date the guidelines are published in the Federal Register.

If your total household income is equal to or higher than the minimum income requirement for your household size, you do not need to provide information on your assets, and you may *not* have a joint sponsor unless you are requested to do so by a Consular or Immigration Officer. If your total household income does not meet the minimum income requirement, the intending immigrant will be ineligible for an immigrant visa or adjustment of status, unless:

- You provide evidence of assets that meet the requirements outlined under "Evidence of Assets" below; and/or

- The immigrant you are sponsoring provides evidence of assets that meet the requirements under "Evidence of Assets" below; or

- A joint sponsor assumes the liability of the intending immigrant with you. A joint sponsor must execute a separate affidavit of support on behalf of the intending

immigrant and any accompanying family members. A joint sponsor must individually meet the minimum requirement of 125 percent of the poverty line based on his or her household size and income and/or assets, including any assets of the sponsored immigrant.

The Government may pursue verification of any information provided on or in support of this form, including employment, income, or assets with the employer, financial or other institutions, the Internal Revenue Service, or the Social Security Administration.

Evidence of Income

In order to complete this form you must submit the following evidence of income:

- A copy of your complete Federal income tax return, as filed with the Internal Revenue Service, for each of the most recent 3 tax years. If you were not required to file a tax return in any of the most recent 3 tax years, you must provide an explanation. If you filed a joint income tax return and are using only your own income to qualify, you must also submit copies of your W-2s for each of the most recent 3 tax years, and if necessary to meet the income requirement, evidence of other income reported on your tax returns, such as Forms 1099.

- If you rely on income of any members of your household or dependents in order to reach the minimum income requirement, copies of their Federal income tax returns for the most recent 3 tax years. These persons must each complete and sign a Form I-864A, Contract Between Sponsor and Household Member.

- Evidence of current employment or self-employment, such as a recent pay statement, or a statement from your employer on business stationery, showing beginning date of employment, type of work performed, and salary or wages paid. You must also provide evidence of current employment for any person whose income is used to qualify.

Evidence of Assets

If you want to use your assets, the assets of your household members or dependents, and/or the assets of the immigrant you are sponsoring to meet the minimum income requirement, you must provide evidence of assets with a cash value that equals at least five times the difference between your total household income and the minimum income requirement. For the assets of a household member, other than the immigrant(s) you are sponsoring, to be considered, the household member must complete and sign Form I-864A, Contract Between Sponsor and Household Member.

All assets must be supported with evidence to verify location, ownership, and value of each asset. Any liens and liabilities relating to the assets must be documented. List only assets that can be readily converted into cash within one year. Evidence of assets includes, but is not limited to the following:

- Bank statements covering the last 12 months, *or a* statement from an officer of the bank or other financial institution in which you have deposits, including deposit/withdrawal history for the last 12 months, and current balance;

- Evidence of ownership and value of stocks, bonds, and certificates of deposit, and date(s) acquired;

- Evidence of ownership and value of other personal property, and date(s) acquired; and

- Evidence of ownership and value of any real estate, and date(s) acquired.

Change of Sponsor's Address

You are required by 8 U.S.C. 1183a(d) and 8 CFR 213a.3 to report every change of address to the Immigration and Naturalization Service and the State(s) in which the sponsored immigrant(s) reside(s). You must report changes of address to INS on Form I-865, Sponsor's Notice of Change of Address, within 30 days of any change of address. You must also report any change in your address to the State(s) in which the sponsored immigrant(s) live.

Penalties

If you include in this affidavit of support any material information that you know to be false, you may be liable for criminal prosecution under the laws of the United States.

If you fail to give notice of your change of address, as required by 8 U.S.C. 1183a(d) and 8 CFR 213a.3, you may be liable for the civil penalty established by 8 U.S.C. 1183a(d)(2). The amount of the civil penalty will depend on whether you failed to give this notice because you were aware that the immigrant(s) you sponsored had received Federal, State, or local means-tested public benefits.

Privacy Act Notice

Authority for the collection of the information requested on this form is contained in 8 U.S.C. 1182(a)(4), 1183a, 1184(a), and 1258. The information will be used principally by the INS or by any Consular Officer to whom it is furnished, to support an alien's application for benefits under the Immigration and Nationality Act and specifically the assertion that he or she has adequate means of financial support and will not become a public charge. Submission of the information is voluntary. Failure to provide the information will result in denial of the application for an immigrant visa or adjustment of status.

The information may also, as a matter of routine use, be disclosed to other Federal, State, and local agencies or private entities providing means-tested public benefits for use in civil action against the sponsor for breach of contract. It may also be disclosed as a matter of routine use to other Federal, State, local, and foreign law enforcement and regulatory agencies to enable these entities to carry out their law enforcement responsibilites.

Reporting Burden

A person is not required to respond to a collection of information unless it displays a currently valid OMB control number. We try to create forms and instructions that are accurate, can be easily understood, and which impose the least possible burden on you to provide us with information. Often this is difficult because some immigration laws are very complex. The reporting burden for this collection of information on Form I-864 is computed as follows: 1) learning about the form, 63 minutes; 2) completing the form, 105 minutes; and 3) assembling and filing the form, 65 minutes, for an estimated average of 3 hours and 48 minutes minutes per response. The reporting burden for collection of information on Form I-864A is computed as: 1) learning about the form, 20 minutes; 2) completing the form, 55 minutes; 3) assembling and filing the form, 30 minutes, for an estimated average of 1 hour and 45 minutes per response. If you have comments regarding the accuracy of this estimates, or suggestions for making this form simpler, you can write to the Immigration and Naturalization Service, HQPDI, 425 I Street, N.W., Room 4034, Washington, DC 20536. **DO NOT MAIL YOUR COMPLETED AFFIDAVIT OF SUPPORT TO THIS ADDRESS.**

CHECK LIST

The following items must be submitted with Form I-864, Affidavit of Support Under Section 213A:

For *ALL* sponsors:

☐ This form, the **I-864, completed and signed** before a notary public or a Consular or Immigration Officer.

☐ Proof of **current employment** or self employment.

☐ Your individual Federal **income tax returns for the most recent 3 tax years,** or an explanation if fewer are submitted. Your **W-2s** for any of the most recent 3 tax years for which you filed a joint tax return that are using only your own income to qualify. Forms 1099 or evidence of other reported income *if* necessary to qualify.

For *SOME* sponsors:

☐ *If the immigrant you are sponsoring is bringing a spouse or children,* **photocopies of the immigrant's affidavit of support** *for each spouse and/or child immigrating with the immigrant you are sponsoring.*

☐ *If you are on active duty in the U.S. Armed Forces and are sponsoring a spouse or child using the 100 percent of poverty level exception,* **proof of your active military status.**

If you are using the income of persons in your household or dependents to qualify,

☐ A separate **Form I-864A** for each person whose income you will use. A sponsored immigrant/household member who is not immigrating with a spouse and/or child **does not need to complete Form I-864A.**

☐ Proof of their **residency and relationship** to you if they are not listed as dependents on your income tax return for the most recent tax year.

☐ Proof of their **current employment** or self-employment.

☐ Copies of their individual Federal **income tax returns for the 3 most recent tax years,** or an explanation if fewer are submitted.

If you use your assets or the assets of the sponsored immigrant to qualify,

☐ **Documentation of assets** establishing location, ownership, date of acquisition, and value. Evidence of any liens or liabilities against these assets.

☐ A separate **Form I-864A** for each household member other than the sponsored immigrant/household member.

If you are a joint sponsor or the relative of an employment-based immigrant requiring an affidavit of support, **proof of your citizenship status.**

☐ For U.S. citizens or nationals, a copy of your birth certificate, passport, or certificate of naturalization or citizenship.

☐ For lawful permanent residents, a copy of both sides of your I-551, Permanent Resident Card.

OMB No. 1115-0214

U.S. Department of Justice
Immigration and Naturalization Service

Affidavit of Support Under Section 213A of the Act

START HERE - Please Type or Print

### Part 1.	Information on Sponsor (You)

Last Name	First Name	Middle Name

Mailing Address *(Street Number and Name)*	Apt/Suite Number

City	State or Province

Country	ZIP/Postal Code	Telephone Number

Place of Residence if different from above *(Street Number and Name)* Apt/Suite Number		**FOR AGENCY USE ONLY**

| City | State or Province |

This Affidavit			Receipt

[ ] Meets

| Country | ZIP/Postal Code | Telephone Number |

[ ] Does not meet

| Date of Birth *(Month, Day, Year)* | Place of Birth *(City, State, Country)* | Are you a U.S. Citizen? ☐ Yes ☐ No |

Requirements of Section 213A

| Social Security Number | A-Number *(If any)* |

### Part 2.	Basis for Filing Affidavit of Support

I am filing this affidavit of support because *(check one)*:

Officer or I.J. Signature

a. ☐	I filed/am filing the alien relative petition.

b. ☐	I filed/am filing an alien worker petition on behalf of the intending

immigrant, who is related to me as my _____ .
							(relationship)

Location

c. ☐	I have ownership interest of at least 5% _____ .
							(name of entity which filed visa petition)

which filed an alien worker petition on behalf of the intending

Date

immigrant, who is related to me as my _____ .
							(relationship)

d. ☐	I am a joint sponsor willing to accept the legal obligations with any other sponsor(s).

### Part 3.	Information on the Immigrant(s) You Are Sponsoring

Last Name	First Name	Middle Name

Date of Birth *(Month,Day, Year)*	Sex ☐ Male ☐ Female	Social Security Number *(If any)*

Country of Citizenship	A-Number *(If any)*

Current Address *(Street Number and Name)*	Apt/Suite Number	City

State/Province	Country	ZIP/Postal Code	Telephone Number

List any spouse and/or children immigrating with the immigrant named above in this Part:		*(Use additional sheet of paper if necessary.)*

Name	Relationship to Sponsored Immigrant			Date of Birth			A-Number *(If any)*	Social Security *(If any)*
	Spouse	Son	Daughter	Mo.	Day	Yr.		

Form I-864 (Rev. 11/05/01)Y

Part 4.   Eligibility to Sponsor

To be a sponsor you must be a U.S. citizen or national or a lawful permanent resident. If you are not the petitioning relative, you must provide proof of status. To prove status, U.S. citizens or nationals must attach a copy of a document proving status, such as a U.S. passport, birth certificate, or certificate of naturalization, and lawful permanent residents must attach a copy of both sides of their Permanent Resident Card (Form I-551).

The determination of your eligibility to sponsor an immigrant will be based on an evaluation of your demonstrated ability to maintain an annual income at or above 125 percent of the Federal poverty line (100 percent if you are a petitioner sponsoring your spouse or child and you are on active duty in the U.S. Armed Forces). The assessment of your ability to maintain an adequate income will include your current employment, household size, and household income as shown on the Federal income tax returns for the 3 most recent tax years. Assets that are readily converted to cash and that can be made available for the support of sponsored immigrants if necessary, including any such assets of the immigrant(s) you are sponsoring, may also be considered.

The greatest weight in determining eligibility will be placed on current employment and household income. If a petitioner is unable to demonstrate ability to meet the stated income and asset requirements, a joint sponsor who *can* meet the income and asset requirements is needed. Failure to provide adequate evidence of income and/or assets or an affidavit of support completed by a joint sponsor will result in denial of the immigrant's application for an immigrant visa or adjustment to permanent resident status.

A. Sponsor's Employment

I am: 1.   ☐ Employed by _____ *(Provide evidence of employment)*

Annual salary _____ or hourly wage $ _____ *(for* _____ *hours per week)*

2.   ☐ Self employed _____ *(Name of business)*

Nature of employment or business _____

3.   ☐ Unemployed or retired since _____

B. Sponsor's Household Size

Number

1. Number of persons (related to you by birth, marriage, or adoption) living in your residence, including yourself *(Do NOT include persons being sponsored in this affidavit.)*   _____

2. Number of immigrants being sponsored in this affidavit *(Include all persons in Part 3.)*   _____

3. Number of immigrants **NOT** living in your household whom you are obligated to support under a previously signed Form I-864.   _____

4. Number of persons who are otherwise dependent on you, as claimed in your tax return for the most recent tax year.   _____

5. Total household size. *(Add lines 1 through 4.)*   **Total**   _____

List persons below who are included in lines 1 or 3 for whom you previously have submitted INS Form I-864, *if your support obligation has not terminated.*

(If additional space is needed, use additional paper)

Name	A-Number	Date Affidavit of Support Signed	Relationship

Part 4.   Eligibility to Sponsor   *(Continued)*

C. Sponsor's Annual Household Income

Enter total unadjusted income from your Federal income tax return for the most recent tax year below. If you last filed a joint income tax return but are using only your *own* income to qualify, list total earnings from your W-2 Forms, or, *if* necessary to reach the required income for your household size, include income from other sources listed on your tax return. If your *individual* income does not meet the income requirement for your household size, you may also list total income for anyone related to you by birth, marriage, or adoption currently living with you in your residence if they have lived in your residence for the previous 6 months, or any person shown as a dependent on your Federal income tax return for the most recent tax year, even if not living in the household. For their income to be considered, household members or dependents must be willing to make their income available for support of the sponsored immigrant(s) and to complete and sign Form I-864A, Contract Between Sponsor and Household Member. A sponsored immigrant/household member only need complete Form I-864A if his or her income will be used to determine your ability to support a spouse and/or children immigrating with him or her.

You must attach evidence of current employment and copies of income tax returns as filed with the IRS for the most recent 3 tax years for yourself and all persons whose income is listed below. See "Required Evidence " in Instructions. Income from all 3 years will be considered in determining your ability to support the immigrant(s) you are sponsoring.

☐   I filed a single/separate tax return for the most recent tax year.
☐   I filed a joint return for the most recent tax year which includes only my own income.
☐   I filed a joint return for the most recent tax year which includes income for my spouse and myself.
    ☐   I am submitting documentation of my individual income (Forms W-2 and 1099).
    ☐   I am qualifying using my spouse's income; my spouse is submitting a Form I-864A.

Indicate most recent tax year   _____
                                                            (tax year)

Sponsor's individual income $_____

or

Sponsor and spouse's combined income $_____
(If spouse's income is to be considered, spouse
must submit Form I-864A.)

Income of other qualifying persons.
(List names; include spouse if applicable.
Each person must complete Form I-864A.)

_____ $_____

_____ $_____

_____ $_____

Total Household Income $_____

Explain on separate sheet of paper if you or any of the above listed individuals were not required to file Federal income tax returns for the most recent 3 years, or if other explanation of income, employment, or evidence is necessary.

D. Determination of Eligibility Based on Income

1. ☐   I am subject to the 125 percent of poverty line requirement for sponsors.
    ☐   I am subject to the 100 percent of poverty line requirement for sponsors on active duty in the U.S. Armed Forces sponsoring their spouse or child.
2. Sponsor's total household size, from Part 4.B., line 5   _____ .
3. Minimum income requirement from the Poverty Guidelines chart for the year of _____ is $ _____
    for this household size.   *(year)*

If you are currently employed and your household income for your household size is equal to or greater than the applicable poverty line requirement (from line D.3.), you do not need to list assets (Parts 4.E. and 5) or have a joint sponsor (Part 6) unless you are requested to do so by a Consular or Immigration Officer. You may skip to Part 7, Use of the Affidavit of Support to Overcome Public Charge Ground of Admissibility. **Otherwise, you should continue with Part 4.E.**

Part 4. Eligibility to Sponsor *(Continued)*

E. Sponsor's Assets and Liabilities

Your assets and those of your qualifying household members and dependents may be used to demonstrate ability to maintain an income at or above 125 percent (or 100 percent, if applicable) of the poverty line *if* they are available for the support of the sponsored immigrant(s) and can readily be converted into cash within 1 year. The household member, other than the immigrant(s) you are sponsoring, must complete and sign Form I-864A, Contract Between Sponsor and Household Member. List the cash value of each asset *after* any debts or liens are subtracted. Supporting evidence must be attached to establish location, ownership, date of acquisition, and value of each asset listed, including any liens and liabilities related to each asset listed. See "Evidence of Assets" in Instructions.

Type of Asset	Cash Value of Assets *(Subtract any debts)*
Savings deposits	$
Stocks, bonds, certificates of deposit	$
Life insurance cash value	$
Real estate	$
Other *(specify)*	$
Total Cash Value of Assets	$ _____

Part 5. Immigrant's Assets and Offsetting Liabilities

The sponsored immigrant's assets may also be used in support of your ability to maintain income at or above 125 percent of the poverty line *if* the assets are or will be available in the United States for the support of the sponsored immigrant(s) and can readily be converted into cash within 1 year.

The sponsored immigrant should provide information on his or her assets in a format similar to part 4.E. above. Supporting evidence must be attached to establish location, ownership, and value of each asset listed, including any liens and liabilities for each asset listed. See "Evidence of Assets" in Instructions.

Part 6. Joint Sponsors

If household income and assets do not meet the appropriate poverty line for your household size, a joint sponsor is required. There may be more than one joint sponsor, but each joint sponsor must individually meet the 125 percent of poverty line requirement based on his or her household income and/or assets, including any assets of the sponsored immigrant. By submitting a separate Affidavit of Support under Section 213A of the Act (Form I-864), a joint sponsor accepts joint responsibility with the petitioner for the sponsored immigrant(s) until they become U.S. citizens, can be credited with 40 quarters of work, leave the United States permanently, or die.

Part 7. Use of the Affidavit of Support to Overcome Public Charge Ground of Inadmissibility

Section 212(a)(4)(C) of the Immigration and Nationality Act provides that an alien seeking permanent residence as an immediate relative (including an orphan), as a family-sponsored immigrant, or as an alien who will accompany or follow to join another alien is considered to be likely to become a public charge and is inadmissible to the United States unless a sponsor submits a legally enforceable affidavit of support on behalf of the alien. Section 212(a)(4)(D) imposes the same requirement on an employment-based immigrant, and those aliens who accompany or follow to join the employment- based immigrant, if the employment-based immigrant will be employed by a relative, or by a firm in which a relative owns a significant interest. Separate affidavits of support are required for family members at the time they immigrate if they are not included on this affidavit of support or do not apply for an immigrant visa or adjustment of status within 6 months of the date this affidavit of support is originally signed. The sponsor must provide the sponsored immigrant(s) whatever support is necessary to maintain them at an income that is at least 125 percent of the Federal poverty guidelines.

> *I submit this affidavit of support in consideration of the sponsored immigrant(s) not being found inadmissible to the United States under section 212(a)(4)(C) (or 212(a)(4)(D) for an employment-based immigrant) and to enable the sponsored immigrant(s) to overcome this ground of inadmissibility. I agree to provide the sponsored immigrant(s) whatever support is necessary to maintain the sponsored immigrant(s) at an income that is at least 125 percent of the Federal poverty guidelines. I understand that my obligation will continue until my death or the sponsored immigrant(s) have become U.S. citizens, can be credited with 40 quarters of work, depart the United States permanently, or die.*

Part 7.   Use of the Affidavit of Support to Overcome Public Charge Grounds   *(Continued)*

Notice of Change of Address.

Sponsors are required to provide written notice of any change of address within 30 days of the change in address until the sponsored immigrant(s) have become U.S. citizens, can be credited with 40 quarters of work, depart the United States permanently, or die. To comply with this requirement, the sponsor must complete INS Form I-865. Failure to give this notice may subject the sponsor to the civil penalty established under section 213A(d)(2) which ranges from $250 to $2,000, unless the failure to report occurred with the knowledge that the sponsored immigrant(s) had received means-tested public benefits, in which case the penalty ranges from $2,000 to $5,000.

> *If my address changes for any reason before my obligations under this affidavit of support terminate, I will complete and file INS Form I-865, Sponsor's Notice of Change of Address, within 30 days of the change of address. I understand that failure to give this notice may subject me to civil penalties.*

Means-tested Public Benefit Prohibitions and Exceptions.

Under section 403(a) of Public Law 104-193 (Welfare Reform Act), aliens lawfully admitted for permanent residence in the United States, with certain exceptions, are ineligible for most Federally-funded means-tested public benefits during their first 5 years in the United States. This provision does not apply to public benefits specified in section 403(c) of the Welfare Reform Act or to State public benefits, including emergency Medicaid; short-term, non-cash emergency relief; services provided under the National School Lunch and Child Nutrition Acts; immunizations and testing and treatment for communicable diseases; student assistance under the Higher Education Act and the Public Health Service Act; certain forms of foster-care or adoption assistance under the Social Security Act; Head Start programs; means-tested programs under the Elementary and Secondary Education Act; and Job Training Partnership Act programs.

Consideration of Sponsor's Income in Determining Eligibility for Benefits.

If a permanent resident alien is no longer statutorily barred from a Federally-funded means-tested public benefit program and applies for such a benefit, the income and resources of the sponsor and the sponsor's spouse will be considered (or deemed) to be the income and resources of the sponsored immigrant in determining the immigrant's eligibility for Federal means-tested public benefits. Any State or local government may also choose to consider (or deem) the income and resources of the sponsor and the sponsor's spouse to be the income and resources of the immigrant for the purposes of determining eligibility for their means-tested public benefits. The attribution of the income and resources of the sponsor and the sponsor's spouse to the immigrant will continue until the immigrant becomes a U.S. citizen or has worked or can be credited with 40 qualifying quarters of work, provided that the immigrant or the worker crediting the quarters to the immigrant has not received any Federal means-tested public benefit during any creditable quarter for any period after December 31, 1996.

> *I understand that, under section 213A of the Immigration and Nationality Act (the Act), as amended, this affidavit of support constitutes a contract between me and the U.S. Government. This contract is designed to protect the United States Government, and State and local government agencies or private entities that provide means-tested public benefits, from having to pay benefits to or on behalf of the sponsored immigrant(s), for as long as I am obligated to support them under this affidavit of support. I understand that the sponsored immigrants, or any Federal, State, local, or private entity that pays any means-tested benefit to or on behalf of the sponsored immigrant(s), are entitled to sue me if I fail to meet my obligations under this affidavit of support, as defined by section 213A and INS regulations.*

Civil Action to Enforce.

If the immigrant on whose behalf this affidavit of support is executed receives any Federal, State, or local means-tested public benefit before this obligation terminates, the Federal, State, or local agency or private entity may request reimbursement from the sponsor who signed this affidavit. If the sponsor fails to honor the request for reimbursement, the agency may sue the sponsor in any U.S. District Court or any State court with jurisdiction of civil actions for breach of contract. INS will provide names, addresses, and Social Security account numbers of sponsors to benefit-providing agencies for this purpose. Sponsors may also be liable for paying the costs of collection, including legal fees.

Part 7. Use of the Affidavit of Support to Overcome Public Charge Grounds *(Continued)*

I acknowledge that section 213A(a)(1)(B) of the Act grants the sponsored immigrant(s) and any Federal, State, local, or private agency that pays any means-tested public benefit to or on behalf of the sponsored immigrant(s) standing to sue me for failing to meet my obligations under this affidavit of support. I agree to submit to the personal jurisdiction of any court of the United States or of any State, territory, or possession of the United States if the court has subject matter jurisdiction of a civil lawsuit to enforce this affidavit of support. I agree that no lawsuit to enforce this affidavit of support shall be barred by any statute of limitations that might otherwise apply, so long as the plaintiff initiates the civil lawsuit no later than ten (10) years after the date on which a sponsored immigrant last received any means-tested public benefits.

Collection of Judgment.

I acknowledge that a plaintiff may seek specific performance of my support obligation. Furthermore, any money judgment against me based on this affidavit of support may be collected through the use of a judgment lien under 28 U.S.C 3201, a writ of execution under 28 U.S.C 3203, a judicial installment payment order under 28 U.S.C 3204, garnishment under 28 U.S.C 3205, or through the use of any corresponding remedy under State law. I may also be held liable for costs of collection, including attorney fees.

Concluding Provisions.

I, _____ , *certify under penalty of perjury under the laws of the United*

States that:

(a) *I know the contents of this affidavit of support signed by me;*

(b) *All the statements in this affidavit of support are true and correct,*

(c) *I make this affidavit of support for the consideration stated in Part 7, freely, and without any mental reservation or purpose of evasion;*

(d) *Income tax returns submitted in support of this affidavit are true copies of the returns filed with the Internal Revenue Service; and*

(e) *Any other evidence submitted is true and correct.*

_____   _____
(Sponsor's Signature)   *(Date)*

Subscribed and sworn to (or affirmed) before me this

_____ day of _____ , _____
                            (Month)   *(Year)*

at _____ .

My commission expires on _____ .

_____
(Signature of Notary Public or Officer Administering Oath)

_____
(Title)

Part 8. If someone other than the sponsor prepared this affidavit of support, that person must complete the following:

I certify under penalty of perjury under the laws of the United States that I prepared this affidavit of support at the sponsor's request, and that this affidavit of support is based on all information of which I have knowledge.

Signature	Print Your Name	Date	Daytime Telephone Number

Firm Name and Address

Index

A

S

About the Author

Brette McWhorter Sember received her J.D. from the State University of New York at Buffalo and practiced in New York state before leaving her practice to become a writer. She is the author of more than twenty books, including how to *Parent with Your Ex: Working Together for Your Child's Best Interest*. She is a member of ASJA (American Society of Journalist and Authors) and AHCJ (Association of Health Care Journalists). She is the recipient of the 1999 Media Award from Family and Home Network (formerly Mothers at Home).

Sember has extensive training in cases involving children and was on the Law Guardian panel in three counties. Her practice included adoptions, which she found to be the happiest cases to take place in Family Court. She is also a trained family mediator and is experienced in a wide variety of family issues. Children have always been her main focus throughout her career.

Sember writes and speaks often about children and family. Her work has appeared in magazines such as *ePregnancy*, *Child*, and *American Baby*. She is the mother of two children and has personal experience with fertility issues.

Your #1 Source for Real World Legal Information...

Sphinx® Publishing
An Imprint of Sourcebooks, Inc.®

- Written by lawyers   • Simple English explanation of the law
  - Forms and instructions included

THE CHILDCARE ANSWER BOOK

With over 80,000 childcare facilities in the US, finding the best childcare solution can be daunting. *The Childcare Answer Book* examines the options available and gives you straightforward, easy-to-use advice on finding the best arrangement that works for you and your child.

304 pages; $12.95;
ISBN 1-57248-482-9

HOW TO PARENT WITH YOUR EX

This manual is the only book designed for both residential and non-residential parents. Formatted and printed in a back-to-back manner as a flip book, it encourages both sides to understand the other's point of view, and so enables both parents to make the most of time spent with the children

376 pages; $16.95;
ISBN 1-57248-479-9

What our customers say about our books:

"It couldn't be more clear for the layperson." —R.D.

"I want you to know I really appreciate your book. It has saved me a lot of time and money." —L.T.

"...many of the legal questions that I have had over the years were answered clearly and concisely through your plain English interpretation of the law." —C.E.H.

"If there weren't people out there like you I'd be lost. You have the best books of this type out there." —S.B.

"...your forms and directions are easy to follow." —C.V.M.

*Sphinx Publishing's Legal Survival Guides are directly available from Sourcebooks, Inc.,
or from your local bookstores. For credit card orders call 1–800–432-7444,
write P.O. Box 4410, Naperville, IL 60567-4410, or fax 630-961-2168*

SPHINX® PUBLISHING'S STATE TITLES

California Titles

How to File for Divorce in CA (5E)	$26.95
How to Settle & Probate an Estate in CA (2E)	$28.95
How to Start a Business in CA (2E)	$21.95
How to Win in Small Claims Court in CA (2E)	$18.95
Landlords' Legal Guide in CA (2E)	$24.95
Make Your Own CA Will	$18.95
Tenants' Rights in CA	$21.95

Florida Titles

Child Custody, Visitation and Support in FL	$26.95
How to File for Divorce in FL (8E)	$28.95
How to Form a Corporation in FL (6E)	$24.95
How to Form a Limited Liability Company in FL (3E)	$24.95
How to Form a Partnership in FL	$22.95
How to Make a FL Will (7E)	$16.95
How to Probate and Settle an Estate in FL (5E)	$26.95
How to Start a Business in FL (7E)	$21.95
How to Win in Small Claims Court in FL (7E)	$18.95
Land Trusts in Florida (7E)	$29.95
Landlords' Rights and Duties in FL (9E)	$22.95

Georgia Titles

How to File for Divorce in GA (5E)	$21.95
How to Start a Business in GA (4E)	$21.95

Illinois Titles

Child Custody, Visitation and Support in IL	$24.95
How to File for Divorce in IL (3E)	$24.95
How to Make an IL Will (3E)	$16.95
How to Start a Business in IL (4E)	$21.95
Landlords' Legal Guide in IL	$24.95

Maryland, Virginia and the District of Columbia Titles

How to File for Divorce in MD, VA, and DC	$28.95
How to Start a Business in MD, VA, or DC	$21.95

Massachusetts Titles

How to Form a Corporation in MA	$24.95
How to Start a Business in MA (4E)	$21.95
Landlords' Legal Guide in MA (2E)	$24.95

Michigan Titles

How to File for Divorce in MI (4E)	$24.95
How to Make a MI Will (3E)	$16.95
How to Start a Business in MI (4E)	$24.95

Minnesota Titles

How to File for Divorce in MN	$21.95
How to Form a Corporation in MN	$24.95
How to Make a MN Will (2E)	$16.95

New Jersey Titles

How to File for Divorce in NJ	$24.95
How to Start a Business in NJ	$21.95

New York Titles

Child Custody, Visitation and Support in NY	$26.95
File for Divorce in NY	$26.95
How to Form a Corporation in NY (2E)	$24.95
How to Make a NY Will (3E)	$16.95
How to Start a Business in NY (3E)	$21.95
How to Win in Small Claims Court in NY (2E)	$18.95
Tenants' Rights in NY	$21.95

North Carolina and South Carolina Titles

How to File for Divorce in NC (3E)	$22.95
How to Make a NC Will (3E)	$16.95
How to Start a Business in NC or SC	$24.95
Landlords' Rights & Duties in NC	$21.95

Ohio Titles

How to File for Divorce in OH (3E)	$24.95
How to Form a Corporation in OH	$24.95
How to Make an OH Will	$16.95

Pennsylvania Titles

Child Custody, Visitation and Support in PA	$26.95
How to File for Divorce in PA (4E)	$26.95
How to Form a Corporation in PA	$24.95
How to Make a PA Will (2E)	$16.95
How to Start a Business in PA (3E)	$21.95
Landlords' Legal Guide in PA	$24.95

Texas Titles

Child Custody, Visitation and Support in TX	$22.95
How to File for Divorce in TX (4E)	$24.95
How to Form a Corporation in TX (3E)	$24.95
How to Probate and Settle an Estate in TX (4E)	$26.95
How to Start a Business in TX (4E)	$21.95
How to Win in Small Claims Court in TX (2E)	$16.95
Landlords' Legal Guide in TX	$24.95
Write Your Own TX Will (4E)	$16.95

Sphinx® Publishing's National Titles

Legal Survival in Business

The Complete Book of Corporate Forms (2E)	$29.95
The Complete Hiring and Firing Handbook	$19.95
The Complete Home-Based Business Kit	$14.95
The Complete Limited Liability Company Kit	$24.95
The Complete Partnership Book	$24.95
The Complete Patent Book	$26.95
The Entrepreneur's Internet Handbook	$21.95
The Entrepreneur's Legal Guide	$26.95
Financing Your Small Business	$17.95
Fired, Laid-Off or Forced Out	$14.95
How to Buy a Franchise	$19.95
How to Form a Nonprofit Corporation (3E)	$24.95
How to Form Your Own (4E) Corporation	$26.95
How to Register Your Own Copyright (5E)	$24.95
HR for Small Business	$14.95
Incorporate in Delaware from Any State	$26.95
Incorporate in Nevada from Any State	$24.95
The Law (In Plain English)® for Small Business	$19.95
The Law (In Plain English)® for Writers	$14.95
Making Music Your Business	$18.95
Minding Her Own Business (4E)	$14.95
Most Valuable Business Legal Forms You'll Ever Need (3E)	$21.95
Profit from Intellectual Property	$28.95
Protect Your Patent	$24.95
The Small Business Owner's Guide to Bankruptcy	$21.95
Tax Power for the Self-Employed	$17.95
Tax Smarts for Small Business	$21.95
Your Rights at Work	$14.95

Legal Survival in Court

Attorney Responsibilities & Client Rights	$19.
Crime Victim's Guide to Justice (2E)	$21.
Legal Research Made Easy (3E)	$21.
Winning Your Personal Injury Claim (3E)	$24.

Legal Survival in Real Estate

The Complete Kit to Selling Your Own Home5	$18.
Essential Guide to Real Estate Contracts (2E)	$18.
Essential Guide to Real Estate Leases	$18.
Homeowner's Rights	$19.
How to Make Money on Foreclosures	$16.
How to Buy a Condominium or Townhome (2E)	$19.
How to Buy Your First Home (2E)	$14.
The Mortgage Answer Book	$14.
The Weekend Landlord	$16.
Working with Your Homeowners Association	$19.

Legal Survival in Spanish

Cómo Comprar su Primera Casa	$8.
Cómo Conseguir Trabajo en los Estados Unidos	$8.
Cómo Hacer su Propio Testamento	$16.
Cómo Negociar su Crédito	$8.
Cómo Organizar un Presupuesto	$8.
Cómo Solicitar su Propio Divorcio	$24.
Guía de Inmigración a Estados Unidos (4E)	$24.
Guía de Justicia para Víctimas del Crimen	$21.
Guía Esencial para los Contratos de Arrendamiento de Bienes Raices	$22.
Inmigración y Ciudadanía en los EE.UU. Preguntas y Respuestas	$16.
Inmigración a los EE.UU. Paso a Paso (2E)	$24.
Manual de Beneficios del Seguro Social	$18.
El Seguro Social Preguntas y Respuestas	$16.
¡Visas! ¡Visas! ¡Visas!	$9.